iNTeROCePTiON
aCTiViTY
aDVeNTURe

Cara Koscinski, OTD, MOT, OTR/L, CAS

iMPoRTanT NoTice

The activities in this book are designed to help understand and strengthen skills for mindfulness, interoception, relaxation, and overall well-being. While these activities can be beneficial, it is important to approach them with care and mindfulness. Kids and adults will benefit from the fun games and ideas presented in this book. All information contained in this book is for educational purposes only. By reading this book, the reader agrees that the author is not responsible for any losses, directly or indirectly, incurred because of the use of the information.

Please keep the following guidelines in mind while practicing any mindfulness or interoceptive activities:

Listen to Your Body:

- Pay close attention to how your body feels during each activity. If you experience any discomfort, dizziness, lightheadedness, or any other adverse symptoms, stop the activity immediately and take a break.

- Do not push yourself beyond your comfort level. Everyone's body is different, and it is important to respect your own limits. Always give kids the opportunity to stop if they feel uncomfortable.

Safe Environment:

- Practice these activities in a safe, comfortable, and quiet environment where you can focus and relax without distractions.

- Ensure that the space around you is free of obstacles to prevent any accidents or injuries.

Medical Conditions:

- If you have any pre-existing medical conditions or health concerns, consult with a healthcare professional before starting any new mindfulness or interoceptive activities.

- Certain activities may not be suitable for individuals with specific health conditions, so it is important to seek professional advice if you are unsure.

Supervision

- An adult should supervise children while practicing these activities to ensure their safety and provide guidance if needed.

- Adults should encourage children to express how they feel during and after the activities and to stop if they feel uncomfortable.

Individual Differences

- Everyone's experience with mindfulness and interoception is unique. What works well for one person may not work for another. It is important to find what feels right for you and to modify activities as needed to suit your individual needs.

Consult Professionals

- If you have any questions or concerns about the activities in this book, consider consulting with a mindfulness coach, therapist, or healthcare professional for personalized guidance and support.

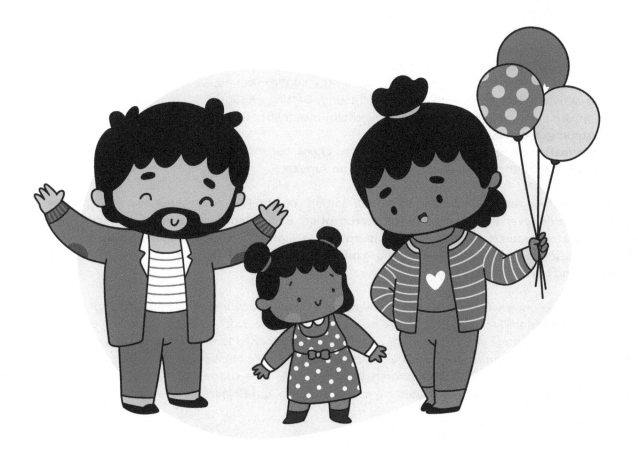

LeT'S exPLoRe ToGeTHeR:
INTRODUCTION TO THE WORKBOOK

I am so excited to help guide you and your child on this incredible journey into the world of interoception! You might be wondering, "What is interoception, and why is it important?" Well, interoception is like having a superpower that helps you understand what is happening inside your body. It also helps you to make sense of your world. Interoception includes the ability to sense your internal body signals, such as hunger, thirst, warmth, cold, and emotions. By tuning into these signals, you can better understand your body and take charge of your health.

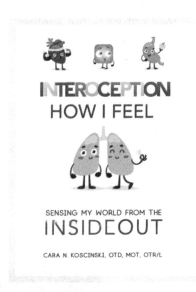

Guess what, your emotions and the way your body feels are linked too! This is why your stomach may have 'butterflies' or tingles when you feel nervous or excited. If you need to present in front of a group, you may begin to sweat or feel your heart pounding. The journey of linking emotions to body signals takes time and the first step is to identify where in the body you're experiencing feelings. Through practice and experience, you begin to make connections and build your own internal vocabulary. Next time you feel stressed, you will learn to recognize the signs before you experience a meltdown. The key is to focus on your internal signals instead of those around you. In this way, you can begin to use mindfulness, breathing, cool-down zones, and other regulating strategies to help increase your comfort. Regulation means being comfortable enough to meet challenges in daily life. We learn best when we are not too tired but not too energetic. It's that 'just right balance.' Interoceptive awareness gives us the superpower to add calming activities to help us with overall well-being. Getting enough oxygen, sleep, drinking water, and engaging in mindfulness activities helps us to understand exactly what our bodies need.

For more information about interoception, be sure to check out my book called, Interoception, How I Feel: Sensing My World from the Inside Out. It's available on Amazon.

In this workbook, you and your child/student will embark on thrilling adventures and engaging activities designed to help discover this superpower of interoception. Each chapter is packed with exciting activities, including games, art projects, role-playing, and journaling, designed to help kids learn in a fun and interactive way. You will also find helpful tips, scientific explanations, and cool facts to deepen understanding of interoception and how it impacts daily life.

The activities in this book will teach and improve interoception for anyone, at any age. Each of the activities is written with child-friendly prompts. They are play-based since the 'work' or occupation of a child is to learn through playing. I encourage you to complete each task with your child to encourage sharing of emotions. All activities have options for groups but can be completed individually. Most of the items throughout the book can be found in your home, office, or classroom. Food activities give suggestions about what specific items are required. Temperature-based tasks need a microwave, stove, or refrigerator/freezer.

How Interoception Develops

When working through activities in this book, keep in mind that developing interoceptive awareness takes a great deal of time and practice, but investing in ourselves always pays off! The first thing we need to do is notice the sensation. For example, if working on toileting, give the child at least 30 seconds to note any changes in the belly like cramping, rumbling, feelings of being full BEFORE using the toilet. Keep track of the feelings DURING the act of pooping or peeing and then, note how it feels AFTER. Look for patterns each time the child uses the toilet to help him to make sense of the body's feelings. The goal is to identify automatic/subconscious information and use it to make conscious decisions. So, when my tummy rumbles, I need to do something. What are my options? I can continue to play, or I can sit on the toilet.

Stages of Interoceptive Awareness

Noticing

Something's happening to my tummy area.

Naming

My tummy feels like its moving or rumbling.

Linking

When my tummy rumbles, I feel hungry.

Understand/Natural Consequence

If I ignore the feeling or rumbling tummy, I get cranky or grumpy.

Managing

Highest level. Stop what I'm doing and take care of issue. I need to eat a snack

Remember, there is no right or wrong way to explore this workbook. Take your time, enjoy the activities, and do not hesitate to revisit chapters and exercises as your child continues to grow and learn. This is your adventure, and every step you take brings you closer to becoming an interoception expert.

So, are you ready to unleash your inner superpower and begin this amazing journey? Let's get started and discover the incredible world inside you!

Dr. Cara Koscinski

iNCLUSiVe aDVeNTURes:
MAKING ACTIVITIES ACCESSIBLE FOR ALL

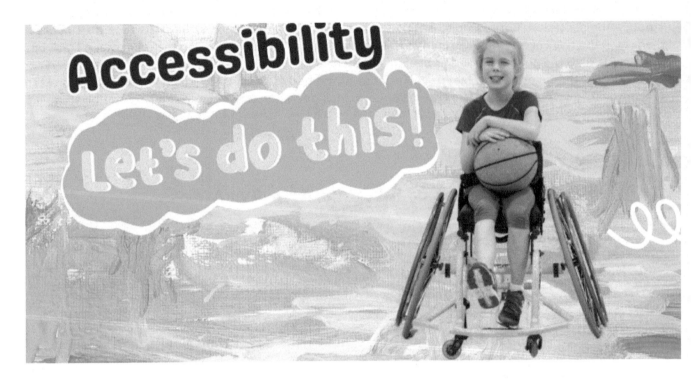

Interoception is a fascinating journey, and it is important that every child, no matter their physical, cognitive, or sensory abilities, can take part in this exploration. Each child has unique needs and preferences, and recognizing these differences allows us to create an environment where everyone feels included, supported, and excited to learn.

Why Adapt Activities?

- **Inclusivity :** Adaptations ensure that all children, regardless of their abilities, can engage in meaningful and enjoyable activities. Inclusivity fosters a sense of belonging and community.

- **Equity :** Providing equal opportunities for all children to participate promotes fairness. It acknowledges that some children may need different approaches to fully engage and learn.

- **Enhanced Learning :** Tailoring activities to meet individual needs can enhance understanding and retention of concepts. It allows children to learn at their own pace and in ways that work best for them.

- **Building Confidence :** When activities are accessible, children are more likely to succeed, which boosts their confidence and encourages further participation.

- **Promoting Empathy :** Inclusive activities teach all children to appreciate and respect differences. They learn to support and celebrate each other's unique strengths and abilities.

Key Considerations for Inclusive Activities

Sensory Preferences : Recognize that some children may be more sensitive to certain textures, sounds, or temperatures. Provide options and allow them to choose what they are comfortable with. We all process sensory information in unique ways, and some may be more or less responsive than others. Sensory processing is also attached to our previous memories and experiences.

Physical Accessibility : Ensure that activities are physically accessible. This might include providing space for wheelchairs, using adaptive tools, or modifying the physical requirements of an activity. Allow children to experience movement in ways that support their comfort level and ability.

Communication Needs : Some children might need visual support, simplified language, or additional time to understand instructions. Be patient and clear in your communication. If children feel uncomfortable or are unable to speak, allow for use of AAC, drawings, and whatever method of communication permits expression.

Behavioral Support : Understand that some children may need additional behavioral support. Create a calm and supportive environment and use positive reinforcement. Never punish a child for not participating or for any emotions arising from the activities. The goal is to help children understand why they might feel this way and how to support their future feelings. It's our job to act as a detective and instead of judging, take time to understand WHY a child might be responding in a certain way. We should adapt the environment for the child's comfort.

Understanding Individual Needs : Begin by understanding the specific needs of each child. This might involve speaking with parents, caregivers, or the children themselves to learn about their preferences, sensitivities, and abilities.

Creating a Flexible Environment : Design activities that can be easily modified. Use flexible materials and open-ended tasks that can be adjusted in complexity and intensity.

Providing Choices : Offer a variety of options for activities. Let children choose materials, tools, or methods that they are most comfortable with.

Using Visual and Sensory Aids : Visual aids, tactile objects, and sensory supports can help children understand and engage with activities. These aids can make instructions clearer and tasks more manageable.

Offering Guidance : Be prepared to provide additional guidance, whether it's through one-on-one assistance, using adaptive tools, or allowing extra time for completion. Patience and encouragement go a long way in making children feel supported.

Adapted Texture Explorations

Description

Modify texture hunts by creating texture boards with a variety of materials (e.g., sandpaper, velvet, bubble wrap) attached to them. Children can feel these textures while sitting or in a comfortable position. Provide a variety of soft and firm objects, like feathers, sponges, and stress balls, and let children choose which ones to touch. Use visual and tactile cues to guide the activity.

- ✓ Use large boards that are easily accessible.
- ✓ Provide a range of textures that are safe and non-irritating.
- ✓ Allow children to explore at their own pace, providing breaks if needed.
- ✓ Offer gloves or a barrier for children who are particularly sensitive to touch.
- ✓ Use simple visual aids to explain textures and associated feelings.

Temperature Activities

Description

Use gel packs that can be heated or cooled to provide safe and controlled temperature experiences. Allow children to touch these packs at their own pace and comfort level. Recognize that sensory processing is different for every child, and some may be sensitive to temperatures. Other children may need more information/input to recognize the sensation.

- ✓ Use cool or warm cloths instead of ice cubes
- ✓ When completing feeding activities, allow the child to test for comfort with temperature
- ✓ Ensure gel packs are not too hot or too cold to avoid discomfort.
- ✓ Provide clear instructions and demonstrations.
- ✓ Allow children to opt-out or use alternative materials if sensitive to temperature changes.
- ✓ Use visual indicators (e.g., color-coded packs) to help children understand temperature differences.
- ✓ Monitor the time children spend with the packs to prevent overstimulation.

Pain Awareness Exploration with Care

Description

Use visual aids and gentle activities to explain the concept of pain. Instead of pinching, use a soft rubber band or a light tap to demonstrate discomfort. Discuss how pain helps protect us.

Goal

Understand the role of nociceptors and the importance of listening to pain signals without causing distress.

- ✓ Use deep breathing exercises during this activity
- ✓ Give positive reinforcement for any attempt
- ✓ Begin with soft items such as feather, cotton ball, soft sponge
- ✓ Play relaxation music in the background

Proprioception and Movement Activities for Everyone

Description

Use stable support (like a wall or chair) for balance activities. Encourage gentle movement exercises like seated yoga or arm stretches to explore proprioception. Allow space for use of wheelchairs or assistive devices. Consider the child's sensitivity to movement against gravity and never force participation.

Goal

Recognize the role of proprioceptors in a safe and supported environment.

Pressure to Skin Activity Choices

Description

Use a variety of objects with different pressures and allow children to choose which ones they want to try. Provide options like soft foam, cotton, cotton swabs, sponges, gentle massage tools, and light weights.

Goal

Understand how mechanoreceptors respond to different pressures with flexible options.

Sensory Storytelling with Supports

Description

Use pictures, tactile books, and simple language to create a sensory story. Encourage children to contribute their sensory experiences and use props to bring the story to life. Sensory experiences are often linked to the child's past experiences and all emotions resulting from sensory activities should be permitted. Provide calming areas or activities for children who need them.

Goal

Enhance descriptive and sensory awareness skills with supportive tools.

Reflection and Journal Activities

Encourage all children to keep a sensation diary, using pictures, drawings, or words. They can note different sensations they experience each day and how they feel about them. Offer alternative methods for journaling, such as using audio recordings or dictation. Permit children to draw pictures, use their preferred AAC method, or any comfortable way to communicate. Consider that new emotions and feelings are being built and encourage children to act without judgement in a safe space.

Supporting Kids with Decreased Verbal Skills

Alternative Communication Methods

- ✓ **Picture Boards :** Use visual aids or picture boards with images representing basic needs, emotions, and activities. Encourage children to point to or select pictures to communicate their thoughts and feelings.

- ✓ **Sign Language :** Introduce simple signs or gestures for commonly used words and phrases. Teach caregivers and peers basic signs to facilitate communication and understanding.

- ✓ **Assistive Communication Devices :** Explore the use of augmentative and alternative communication (AAC) devices, such as speech-generating devices or communication apps. These tools can provide voice output for children who have difficulty speaking.

Non-Verbal Communication Strategies

Gestures : Encourage the use of gestures and body language to convey messages. Teach children simple gestures for common needs or actions, such as pointing to indicate a desired object or raising their hand to ask for help.

Facial Expressions : Pay attention to facial expressions as a means of communication. Children may use facial expressions to express emotions, preferences, or discomfort. Respond sensitively to their cues to facilitate understanding and connection.

Visual Supports and Cues

Visual Schedules : Create visual schedules or timetables to provide structure and predictability. Use pictures or symbols to represent daily routines, activities, and transitions. Refer to the schedule regularly to help children anticipate and understand upcoming events.

Visual Choice Boards : Offer visual choice boards with pictures or symbols representing different options. Use these boards to allow children to make choices about activities, snacks, or preferred items. This empowers them to express their preferences and make decisions independently.

Encouraging Participation and Engagement

Active Listening : Practice active listening by giving children your full attention and acknowledging their attempts to communicate. Respond with patience, encouragement, and positive reinforcement to build confidence and trust.

Creating Opportunities for Interaction : Facilitate opportunities for children to engage in social interactions and activities with peers. Encourage inclusive play and communication by pairing children with similar interests and abilities.

Modeling Communication : Model effective communication strategies by using clear and simple language, gestures, and visual supports. Encourage imitation and participation by demonstrating how to use alternative communication methods in various contexts.

Collaboration with Caregivers and Professionals:

Family Involvement : Collaborate closely with caregivers to understand each child's unique communication needs, preferences, and strategies. Provide resources, training, and support to help caregivers implement communication strategies at home.

Multidisciplinary Support : Seek input and collaboration from speech-language pathologists, special education teachers, occupational therapists, and other professionals with expertise in communication and assistive technology. Together, develop individualized plans and strategies to support children's communication development and participation.

Creating a Supportive Environment:

Patience and Understanding : Be patient and understanding when communicating with children with decreased verbal skills. Allow them time to process information and respond at their own pace. Avoid rushing or pressuring them to communicate verbally.

Respect and Dignity : Treat children with respect and dignity, recognizing their inherent value and worth. Validate their communication attempts and efforts, regardless of the form or modality used. Foster a supportive and inclusive environment where all forms of communication are valued and accepted.

By implementing these strategies and providing a supportive and inclusive environment, we can empower children with decreased verbal skills to communicate effectively, participate actively, and engage meaningfully in the world around them.

Creating an inclusive environment ensures that all children can explore and benefit from the wonders of interoception. By adapting activities to meet diverse needs, we can make sure that everyone has the opportunity to learn, grow, and enjoy the journey. Keep exploring, supporting one another, and celebrating the unique ways we all experience the world!

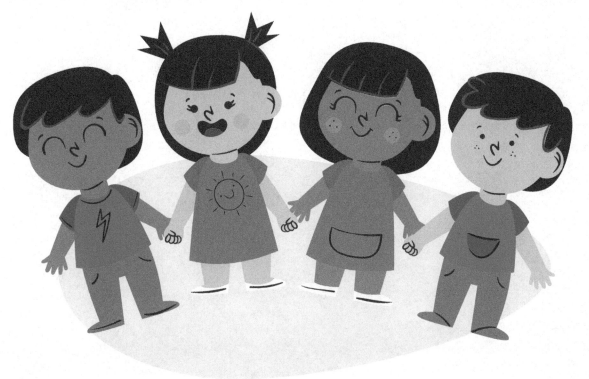

CHAPTER - 1

UNLEASH YOUR SUPERPOWER

Interoception Explorers

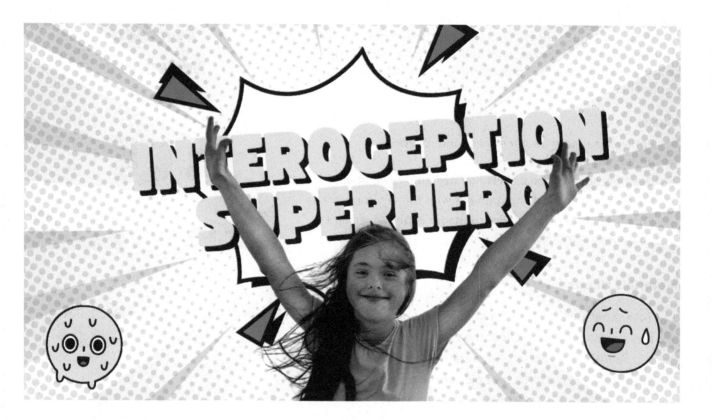

In this chapter, children embark on an exhilarating adventure to discover their inner superpower: interoception. Interoception allows us to sense what is happening inside our bodies, like feeling hungry or thirsty. Interoception, a lesser-known sense, involves sensing signals from inside the body, such as heartbeat, hunger, or fatigue. These signals are transmitted through nerves in the body, particularly the vagus nerve, and processed in the brain's insular cortex. Through fun activities and explorations, children will learn to recognize and understand their body's signals, empowering them to take control of their well-being.

Sensory Sensation Safari Activities

Sensory Scavenger Expedition

Overview : Embark on a thrilling scavenger hunt around the house, classroom, or outside to find different items that relate to the eight senses (sight, hearing, touch, taste, smell, proprioceptive, vestibular, and interoception). This activity will help children connect physical sensations to their sensory experiences.

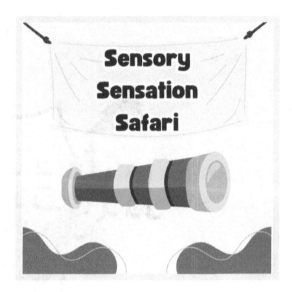

Goals

- ✓ Enhance sensory awareness and interoceptive understanding.
- ✓ Develop observational skills and descriptive abilities.
- ✓ Foster curiosity and engagement with the environment.
- ✓ Encourage discussions about sensory experiences and emotional responses.

Materials Needed

- ✓ Scavenger Hunt List : A list of items to find that correspond to each of the senses. Provided below.
- ✓ Bags or Baskets : To collect the items found during the hunt.
- ✓ Notebooks and Pencils : For noting observations and feelings.
- ✓ Camera (Optional) : To take pictures of the items found.

Instructions

Preparation : Create a scavenger hunt list with items related to each of the eight senses. Here are some examples:

- ✓ **Sight :** A colorful flower, a shiny object, a favorite toy.
- ✓ **Hearing :** A bird singing, a musical instrument, a ticking clock.
- ✓ **Touch :** Something soft (like a stuffed animal), something rough (like sandpaper), something smooth (like a stone).
- ✓ **Taste :** A piece of fruit, a salty snack, a sweet treat.
- ✓ **Smell :** A scented candle, a flower, a spice from the kitchen.
- ✓ **Proprioceptive :** An item that involves pushing or pulling (like a door), something heavy to lift (like a small weight), or something to squeeze (like a stress ball).
- ✓ **Vestibular :** An item that can spin or swing (like a hula hoop or a swing), something to balance on (like a balance board), or an item that rolls (like a ball).
- ✓ **Interoceptive :** An item that brings excitement, happiness, or joy

Explaining the Hunt

Explain the purpose of the scavenger hunt: to find items that relate to the eight senses and explore how each item makes them feel. Discuss safety rules and boundaries, especially if the hunt takes place outside.

Starting the Expedition

Give each child a scavenger hunt list, a bag or basket to collect items, and a notebook and pencil. Set a time limit for the scavenger hunt to add excitement.

Finding and Collecting Items

Children should find and collect items from the list that match each of the senses. Encourage them to use their senses actively as they search for each item (e.g., listening carefully for sounds, feeling textures, engaging in movement).

Observing and Recording

Once all items are found, gather the children to discuss their discoveries. Ask them to observe each item closely and note their observations in their notebooks. For example:

✓ What does the item look like?

✓ What sound does it make?

✓ How does it feel to touch?

✓ What does it taste like (for taste-safe items)?

✓ What does it smell like?

✓ How does it feel to move with or around the item (proprioceptive and vestibular)?

Discussing Feelings and Body Sensations : Have a group discussion about how each item makes them feel and where they feel it in their bodies. Ask questions such as:

✓ How does this item make you feel?

✓ Do you feel happy, excited, relaxed, or something else?

✓ Where do you feel this sensation in your body? (e.g., butterflies in the stomach, a warm feeling in the chest).

✓ How do movements make your body feel? (e.g., balanced, dizzy, strong).

Recording Feelings

In their notebooks, children can draw or write about their feelings and the corresponding body sensations for each item.

Sharing and Reflecting

Encourage children to share their favorite discoveries and describe their sensory experiences. Reflect on the importance of paying attention to sensory signals and how they help us understand our environment and motions.

Conclusion : The Sensory Scavenger Expedition is a fun and interactive way to help children connect their sensory experiences with their body sensations and emotions. By exploring and discussing these connections, children can develop a deeper understanding of how their bodies respond to different stimuli and enhance their interoceptive awareness.

Feelings Mosaic Madness: An Exciting Texture Adventure

Feelings Mosaic Madness is an engaging and creative activity designed to help children express their emotions and understand the complex nature of feelings through art. This adventure allows kids to create a mosaic that represents different emotions using assorted colors and materials, making it a fun and therapeutic experience.

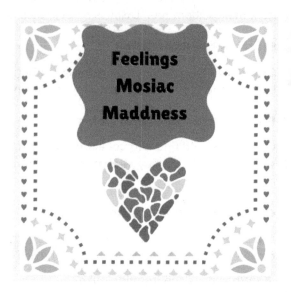

Goals

✓ Enhance emotional literacy by associating colors and textures with different feelings.

✓ Foster creativity and self-expression through art.

✓ Encourage discussions about emotions and their physical manifestations.

✓ Develop fine motor skills and hand-eye coordination.

Materials Needed

✓ Colored Paper : Assorted colors representing different emotions (e.g., yellow for happiness, blue for sadness, red for anger, green for calm, purple for excitement). Encourage the child to choose colors to represent the emotions. If you use the any formal programs such as Zones of Regulation, use the same colors for consistency.

✓ Textured Materials : Felt, fabric scraps, sandpaper, cotton balls, scrapbooking supplies, tissue paper, and more to add a tactile element to the mosaic.

✓ Scissors and Glue : Safe scissors for cutting and glue sticks or liquid glue for assembling the mosaic.

✓ Large Poster Board or Canvas : A base for the mosaic.

✓ Markers or Crayons : For drawing outlines and adding details.

✓ Emotion Cards : Small cards with different emotional words and associated facial expressions to guide the activity. Cards are provided in the resources section at the end of this book. Whenever possible, when teaching emotions, it is best to take actual photos of the child's face as he acts out the emotion.

Instructions

✓ Introduction : Begin by discussing the different emotions and how they can be represented through colors and textures. Show examples of how colors can symbolize different feelings (e.g., red for anger, blue for sadness).

✓ Select Emotions : Allow each child to choose a few emotions they want to represent in their mosaic. They can use emotion cards for inspiration.

✓ Choose Colors and Textures : Have the children select colored paper and textured materials that they feel best represent the chosen emotions. Explain how different textures can also symbolize feelings (e.g., soft cotton for comfort, rough sandpaper for frustration).

✓ **Create Mosaic Pieces** : Guide the children to cut the colored paper and textured materials into small pieces or shapes. These pieces will be used to create the mosaic.

✓ **Design the Mosaic** : Encourage children to arrange their pieces on the poster board or canvas to form patterns or images that express their emotions. They can draw outlines of shapes or pictures to fill in with the mosaic pieces.

✓ **Assemble the Mosaic** : Help the children glue the pieces onto the poster board or canvas. Encourage them to think about how the placement of each piece and the combination of colors and textures convey their feelings.

Discussion

Once the mosaics are complete, have a group discussion where each child explains their artwork and the emotions they represent. Ask questions like:
✓ Why did you choose these colors and textures?
✓ How do these colors make you feel?
✓ Can you describe a time when you felt this way?

Display the Artwork

Create a gallery space to display the completed mosaics. This can be a wall in the classroom or a designated area at home. Encourage children to share their work with family and friends.

Turn Activity 2 into an Adventurous Journey: Emotion Adventure Map

Turn the activity into an adventurous journey by creating an **"Emotion Adventure Map."** Each child starts at a specific emotion on the map and travels through different emotional "lands," adding to their mosaic as they go. By combining creativity with emotional learning, "Emotion Adventure Map" becomes an exciting activity that not only entertains but also educates and empowers children to understand and express their emotions.

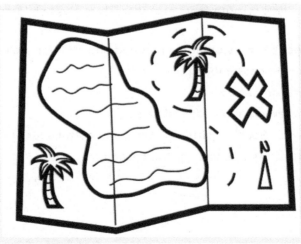

Benefits

✓ Emotional Expression : Provides a safe and creative outlet for expressing complex emotions.

✓ Empathy and Understanding : Helps children understand their own emotions and those of others by seeing different interpretations.

✓ Artistic Skills : Enhances artistic abilities and appreciation for visual arts.

✓ Communication : Promotes verbal expression and storytelling as children explain their artwork.

Feelings Fiesta Collage:

Overview

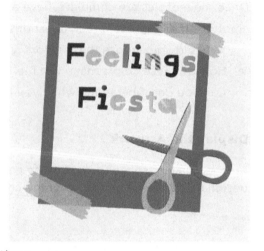

The Feelings Fiesta Collage is a creative and interactive activity designed to help children explore and express their emotions through art. By using a variety of materials and images, children will create a collage that represents their feelings, promoting emotional awareness and self-expression.

Goals

✓ Enhance emotional literacy by identifying and expressing feelings.
✓ Foster creativity and artistic skills.
✓ Encourage discussions about emotions and their physical sensations.
✓ Develop fine motor skills and hand-eye coordination.

Materials Needed

✓ Magazines and Newspapers : For cutting out images and words.
✓ Comic Strips or using the child's favorite fonts and characters gives children a sense of excitement and agency during the activity.
✓ Colored Paper and Cardstock : For a vibrant background and additional elements.
✓ Glue Sticks and Liquid Glue : For assembling the collage.
✓ Scissors : Child-safe scissors for cutting.
✓ Markers and Crayons : For drawing and adding details.
✓ Stickers and Decorative Items : Such as glitter, sequins, and buttons for embellishment.
✓ Large Poster Board or Canvas : As the base for the collage.

Instructions

Begin by discussing different emotions and how they can be expressed through art. Show examples of collages and explain the concept of using images, colors, and words to represent feelings.

✅ Choosing Emotions :

Ask each child to think about a few emotions they have recently felt or want to explore. Provide emotion cards or a list of feelings (e.g., happy, sad, excited, nervous, calm) to help them choose. Emotions cards can be found in the resources section at the back of this book.

✅ Gathering Materials :

✓ Distribute magazines, newspapers, colored paper, and other decorative items.
✓ Encourage children to cut out images, words, and shapes that they feel represent their chosen emotions.

✅ Creating the Collage :

✓ Give each child a large poster board or canvas as their base.
✓ Have them arrange and glue the cut-out images, words, and shapes onto the base to create their collage.
✓ Encourage them to use colors and textures that match their feelings (e.g., bright colors for happiness, cool colors for calmness).

✅ Adding Personal Touches :

Provide markers, crayons, and additional decorative items for children to add personal touches to their collages. They can draw, write, or add stickers and other embellishments to enhance their artwork.

✅ Reflecting and Sharing :

✓ Once the collages are complete, gather the children to share their creations.
✓ Ask each child to explain their collage, discussing the images, colors, and words they chose and what emotions they represent.
✓ Encourage them to talk about how these emotions feel in their bodies and any physical sensations they associate with them.

✅ Discussion Questions :

✓ What emotions did you choose to represent in your collage?
✓ How do the colors and images you selected relate to your feelings?
✓ Can you describe a time when you felt one of these emotions?
✓ Where in your body do you feel these emotions?

✅ Benefits :

✓ Emotional Expression: Provides a safe and creative outlet for expressing complex emotions.
✓ Empathy and Understanding: Helps children understand their own emotions and those of others by seeing different interpretations.
✓ Artistic Skills: Enhances artistic abilities and appreciation for visual arts.
✓ Communication : Promotes verbal expression and storytelling as children explain their artwork.

Conclusion : The Feelings Fiesta Collage is a fun and engaging activity that allows children to explore their emotions through art. By creating and discussing their collages, children can develop a deeper understanding of their feelings and learn to express them in a healthy and creative way.

Body Awareness Safari

Overview

The Body Awareness Safari is an interactive and engaging activity designed to help children explore and understand their body's movements and sensations. By mimicking different animal movements and paying attention to how their bodies feel, children will enhance their proprioceptive and interoceptive awareness.

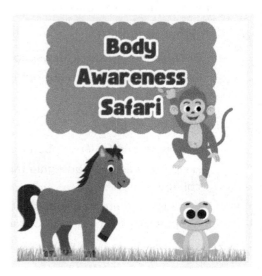

Goals

✓ Improve body awareness and coordination.

✓ Enhance proprioceptive and interoceptive skills.

✓ Foster creativity and physical activity.

✓ Encourage discussions about how different movements make their bodies feel.

Materials Needed

✓ Open Space : A safe area indoors or outdoors where children can move freely.

✓ Animal Cards : Animal cards can be found in the resources section at the back of this book.

✓ Music (Optional) : Upbeat music to add excitement and rhythm to the activity.

✓ Notebooks and Pencils : For noting observations and feelings.

✓ Props (Optional) : Items like scarves, hoops, or small obstacles to enhance animal movements.

Instructions

✓ Explain the concept of a safari and how explorers observe animals in their natural habitats.

✓ Introduce the idea of mimicking animal movements to understand how different parts of the body work.

  ✓ Animal Movements : Show the animal cards to the children and explain the movements associated with each animal. Examples include:

- Lion : Crawling on all fours and stretching.
- Kangaroo : Hopping with both feet together.
- Elephant : Stomping with heavy steps and swinging an arm like a trunk.
- Horse : Gallop, trot, prance.
- Butterfly : Flapping arms gently as wings.
- Giraffe : Walking on tiptoes with arms extended overhead.

- Crab : Walking sideways on hands and feet.
- Frog : Squatting and jumping forward.
- Cheetah : Sprinting with short bursts of speed
- Bird : Flap arms like wings.
- Starfish : Stretch out arms and legs slowly and hold
- Snake : Lay on ground, prone and slither on the floor forward with arms in wiggling motion.

✓ Starting the Safari:

✓ Designate an area as the safari zone where children will perform the animal movements.

✓ Play music if desired to create a fun and lively atmosphere.

✓ Exploring Movements: Call out an animal and demonstrate its movement. Encourage the children to mimic the movement and pay attention to how their bodies feel. Rotate through different animals, allowing each child to experience a variety of movements.

Observing and Recording

✓ After each movement, pause and ask the children how their bodies feel. Questions to consider include:

✓ Which muscles are you using?

✓ How does your heart feel?

✓ Are you breathing faster?

✓ Do you feel balanced or wobbly?

✓ Have children note their observations and feelings in their notebooks.

Adding Props (Optional)

Introduce props to make the movements more engaging. For example:

✓ Use scarves for butterfly wings.

✓ Set up small obstacles for kangaroos to hop over.

✓ Provide hoops for lions to crawl through.

Group Discussion

✓ After the safari, gather the children to discuss their experiences. Ask questions like:

✓ Which animal movement was your favorite and why?

✓ Which movement was the most challenging?

✓ How did different movements make your body feel?

✓ Can you think of other animals and how they move?

Reflecting on Body Awareness : Talk about the importance of body awareness and how it helps us in everyday activities, such as sports, dancing, and even sitting comfortably. Encourage children to practice body awareness in other activities throughout the day.

Benefits

✓ Physical Activity : Promotes exercise and helps develop gross motor skills.

✓ Body Awareness : Enhances understanding of how different parts of the body work together.

✓ Proprioception : Improves the ability to sense body position and movement.

✓ Interoception : Encourages noticing internal body signals like heartbeat and muscle tension.

✓ Creativity : Fosters imaginative play and creative thinking.

Conclusion : The Body Awareness Safari is a fun and educational activity that helps children connect with their bodies through movement and play. By mimicking different animal movements, children can develop a deeper understanding of their body's capabilities and sensations, enhancing both proprioceptive and interoceptive awareness.

Yoga Journey

Objective

To promote relaxation, flexibility, and body awareness through yoga poses inspired by nature and animals.

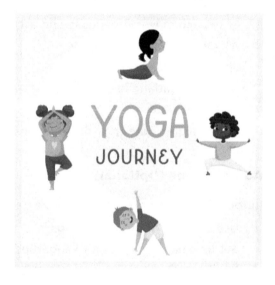

Materials Needed

✓ Yoga mat or comfortable space

✓ Drawing paper and markers

✓ Comfortable clothing

Goals

✓ Enhance body awareness and mindfulness

✓ Improve balance, flexibility, and strength

✓ Promote relaxation and reduce stress

✓ Encourage creativity and self-expression

✓ Foster a routine of physical activity and mental well-being

How to Complete

✓ Learn Poses : Learn various yoga poses inspired by nature and animals. Use online resources, books, or yoga cards to find poses that interest you.

✓ Create a Routine : Design a yoga routine with your favorite poses. Draw or write about each pose and its benefits.

✓ Practice : Practice your yoga routine, focusing on your breathing and how each pose makes your body feel.

✓ Reflect : Think about how your body feels after the yoga session. Do you feel more relaxed, flexible, or balanced?

✓ Share : Share your yoga routine with family or friends and practice together.

Yoga Poses to Include

✓ Tree Pose (Vrksasana) : Stand on one leg, place the sole of the other foot on the inner thigh or calf, and raise your arms above your head. This pose improves balance and focus.

✓ Mountain Pose (Tadasana) : Stand tall with feet together, arms at your sides, and palms facing forward. This pose promotes good posture and grounding.

✓ Cat-Cow Stretch (Marjaryasana-Bitilasana) : On hands and knees, alternate between arching your back (cow) and rounding it (cat). This pose increases flexibility in the spine.

✓ Downward-Facing Dog (Adho Mukha Svanasana) : From a plank position, lift your hips up and back, forming an inverted V-shape. This pose stretches the back, legs, and shoulders.

✓ Butterfly Pose (Baddha Konasana) : Sit with your feet together and knees bent out to the sides. Hold your feet and gently flap your legs like butterfly wings. This pose opens the hips.

✓ Child's Pose (Balasana) : Sit back on your heels, stretch your arms forward, and lower your forehead to the mat. This pose promotes relaxation and stretches the back.

✓ Cobra Pose (Bhujangasana) : Lie on your stomach, place your hands under your shoulders, and lift your chest off the ground. This pose strengthens the back and opens the chest.

✓ Warrior I (Virabhadrasana I) : Step one foot forward into a lunge, turn the back foot slightly out, and raise your arms overhead. This pose builds strength and stability.

✓ Warrior II (Virabhadrasana II) : From Warrior I, open your hips and arms to the side, gazing over your front hand. This pose enhances strength and concentration.

✓ Triangle Pose (Trikonasana) : Stand with your feet wide apart, turn one foot out, and reach your arm down to the ankle while extending the other arm up. This pose stretches the sides and improves balance.

✓ Bridge Pose (Setu Bandhasana) : Lie on your back with knees bent, lift your hips towards the ceiling, and clasp your hands under your back. This pose strengthens the back and legs.

✓ Seated Forward Bend (Paschimottanasana) : Sit with legs extended, reach forward, and try to touch your toes. This pose stretches the back and hamstrings.

✓ Happy Baby Pose (Ananda Balasana) : Lie on your back, bend your knees, and hold the outside edges of your feet. This pose opens the hips and relaxes the lower back.

✓ Pigeon Pose (Kapotasana) : From a plank position, bring one knee forward and extend the other leg back, lowering your hips. This pose stretches the hips and thighs.

✓ Plank Pose : Hold a push-up position with your body in a straight line. This pose strengthens the core and upper body.

✓ Boat Pose (Navasana) : Sit with your legs extended, lean back slightly, and lift your legs off the ground, balancing on your sit bones. This pose strengthens the core.

✓ Eagle Pose (Garudasana) : Stand on one leg, wrap the other leg around it, and cross your arms in front of you. This pose improves balance and stretches the shoulders.

✓ Fish Pose (Matsyasana) : Lie on your back, arch your chest up, and place the crown of your head on the mat. This pose opens the chest and throat.

✓ Lizard Pose (Utthan Pristhasana) : From a plank position, bring one foot forward outside your hand and lower your hips. This pose stretches the hips and legs.

✓ Savasana (Corpse Pose) : Lie flat on your back, arms at your sides, and close your eyes. This pose promotes deep relaxation and mindfulness.

Detailed Yoga Journey Routine

- Warm-Up: Mountain Pose and Cat-Cow Stretch
  - ✓ Mountain Pose (Tadasana) : Stand tall with feet together, arms at your sides, and palms facing forward. Take deep breaths, feeling the ground beneath your feet.
  - ✓ Cat-Cow Stretch (Marjaryasana-Bitilasana) : On hands and knees, alternate between arching your back (cow) and rounding it (cat). Inhale as you arch and exhale as you round.

- Balance and Strength: Tree Pose and Warrior I
  - ✓ Tree Pose (Vrksasana) : Stand on one leg, place the sole of the other foot on the inner thigh or calf, and raise your arms above your head. Hold for a few breaths, then switch sides.
  - ✓ Warrior I (Virabhadrasana I) : Step one foot forward into a lunge, turn the back foot slightly out, and raise your arms overhead. Hold for a few breaths, then switch sides.

- Flexibility and Stretching: Downward-Facing Dog and Butterfly Pose
  - ✓ Downward-Facing Dog (Adho Mukha Svanasana): From a plank position, lift your hips up and back, forming an inverted V-shape. Hold for a few breaths.
  - ✓ Butterfly Pose (Baddha Konasana) : Sit with your feet together and knees bent out to the sides. Hold your feet and gently flap your legs like butterfly wings.

- Relaxation and Mindfulness: Child's Pose and Savasana
  - ✓ Child's Pose (Balasana): Sit back on your heels, stretch your arms forward, and lower your forehead to the mat. Hold for a few breaths.
  - ✓ Savasana (Corpse Pose) : Lie flat on your back, arms at your sides, and close your eyes. Focus on your breathing and let your body relax completely.

Reflection and Sharing

After completing your Yoga Journey routine, take a few moments to reflect on how your body feels. Use drawing paper and markers to draw or write about your experience. Consider the following questions:

✓ How did each pose make your body feel?

✓ Which poses did you enjoy the most?

✓ How do you feel now compared to before the yoga session?

Share your reflections and drawings with family or friends and encourage them to join you on your next Yoga Journey.

By engaging in these Yoga Journey activities, you will enhance your body awareness, improve your balance and flexibility, and promote relaxation. Enjoy these fun yoga poses and explore the wonderful benefits of movement and mindfulness!

Proprioceptive Play Activities

Balance Challenge Adventure
Objective

To enhance balance, coordination, and body awareness through various proprioceptive activities.

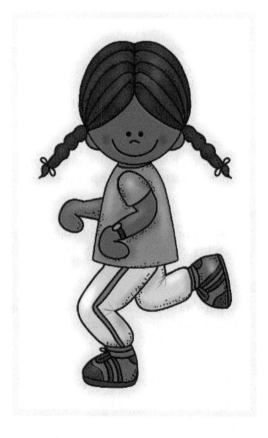

Materials Needed

✓ Open space for movement

✓ Timer

✓ Drawing paper and markers

✓ Comfortable clothing

Goals

✓ Improve balance and coordination

✓ Increase body awareness

✓ Promote physical activity and fun

✓ Encourage self-reflection and mindfulness

✓ Develop a sense of achievement and confidence

How to Complete

✓ Introduction to Proprioception : Explain that proprioception is your body's ability to sense its position and movement in space. Activities that challenge balance and coordination can help improve this sense.

✓ Warm-Up Activities : Start with a few simple warm-up exercises to get your body ready. These can include marching in place, arm circles, and gentle stretching.

✓ Balance Challenge Stations : Set up different stations for various balance and proprioceptive activities. Rotate through each station, spending a few minutes at each.

Balance Challenge Stations

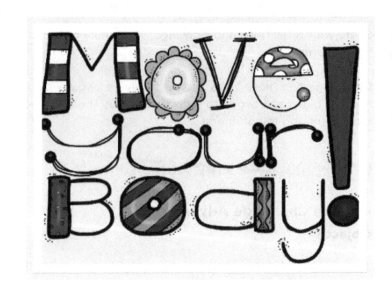

- ✅ **One-Foot Stand**

  Stand on one foot and try to maintain your balance for as long as possible. Switch to the other foot and repeat. Use a timer to track how long you can balance on each foot.

- ✅ **Heel-to-Toe Walk**

  Walk in a straight line, placing the heel of one foot directly in front of the toes of the other foot. Try to walk as smoothly and steadily as possible.

- ✅ **Balance Beam Walk**

  Use a piece of tape or a narrow board to create a balance beam on the floor. Walk along the beam, focusing on keeping your balance.

- ✅ **Tree Pose**

  Stand on one leg, place the sole of the other foot on the inner thigh or calf, and raise your arms above your head. Hold the pose for several breaths, then switch sides.

- ✅ **Bean Bag Balance**

  Place a bean bag or small object on your head and try to walk around without letting it fall. This activity challenges your balance and coordination.

- ✅ **Obstacle Course**

  Create a simple obstacle course using household items like pillows, chairs, and boxes. Include activities that require crawling, jumping, and balancing.

- ✅ **Bouncing Ball**

  Stand on one foot while bouncing a ball against a wall and catching it. Switch to the other foot and repeat.

- ✅ **Chair Pose**

  Stand with your feet together, bend your knees, and lower your hips as if you are sitting in an invisible chair. Hold the pose for several breaths.

- ✅ **Lunges**

  Step forward with one leg and lower your body until both knees are bent at a 90-degree angle. Push back up to the starting position and switch legs.

- Star Jumps

    Jump up and spread your arms and legs out like a star, then land back in the starting position. Repeat several times.

- Reflect and Draw
    - After completing the balance challenges, take a few moments to reflect on how your body felt during each activity. Use drawing paper and markers to draw or write about your experience.
    - Consider the following questions:
        - Which balance activity was the most challenging?
        - How did your body feel during and after the activities?
        - Did you notice any improvements in your balance and coordination?

- Share Your Experience
    - Share your drawings and reflections with family or friends. Discuss which activities you enjoyed the most and why.
    - Encourage others to join you in your balance challenges and see how they do!

By engaging in these Balance Challenge Adventure activities, you will enhance your body awareness, improve your balance and coordination, and have fun exploring the wonderful world of proprioception. Enjoy these activities and feel confident in your ability to navigate your body in space!

Body Mapping Voyage

Chart the course of your body sensations on a large piece of paper. With different colored markers, draw or write about where you feel certain sensations when you are hungry, thirsty, tired, or happy. Discuss your body map with others and compare similarities and differences.

Body Mapping

Overview

The Body Mapping Voyage is a creative and introspective activity that allows children to chart the course of their body sensations on a large piece of paper. Using different colored markers, they can draw or write about where they feel certain sensations when they experience various emotions or physical states, such as hunger, thirst, tiredness, or happiness. This activity encourages self-awareness and provides a visual representation of interoceptive signals.

Goals

- Enhance interoceptive awareness by identifying and mapping body sensations.
- Promote self-expression and creativity.
- Foster discussions about personal experiences and bodily awareness.
- Develop fine motor skills and the ability to articulate internal experiences.

Materials Needed

✓ Large Sheets of Paper : Big enough to accommodate a full-body outline.

✓ Colored Markers : Different colors to represent various sensations and emotions.

✓ Body Outline Templates (Optional) : Pre-drawn outlines of a body for children to use as a guide.

✓ Notebooks and Pencils : For noting observations and reflections.

✓ Stickers or Decorative Items (Optional) : To enhance the body maps.

Instructions

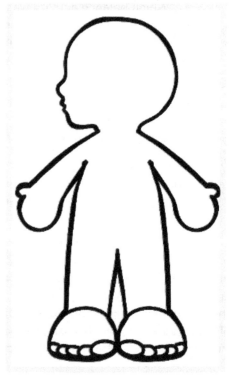

- Explain the concept of body mapping and how it can help visualize where we feel different sensations and emotions in our bodies.

- Discuss common body sensations associated with emotions and physical states, such as feeling butterflies in the stomach when nervous or a warm feeling in the chest when happy.

- Creating the Body Map

  ✓ Provide each child with a large sheet of paper and colored markers If using templates, give them the pre-drawn body outlines.

  ✓ Have each child lie down on their paper while a partner traces their body outline with a marker. Alternatively, use the pre-drawn outlines.

- Identifying Sensations

  ✓ Ask the children to think about where they feel certain sensations in their bodies during different states: **Allow the child to use descriptive language

  ✓ Hunger : Where do you feel hunger in your body? (e.g., stomach growling, empty feeling in the belly)

  ✓ Thirst : Where do you feel thirst? (e.g., dry throat, mouth feeling parched)

  ✓ Tiredness : Where do you feel tiredness? (e.g., heavy eyelids, sluggish limbs)

  ✓ Happiness : Where do you feel happiness? (e.g., warm feeling in the chest, lightness in the body)

  ✓ Nervousness : Where do you feel nervousness? (e.g., butterflies in the stomach, sweaty palms)

  ✓ Excitement : Where do you feel excitement? (e.g., quickened heartbeat, tingling in the fingers)

  ✓ Anger : Where do you feel anger? (e.g., tightness in the fists, heat in the face)

  ✓ Sadness : Where do you feel sadness? (e.g., heavy chest, tears in the eyes)

  ✓ Calmness : Where do you feel calmness? (e.g., relaxed muscles, slow, deep breaths)

  ✓ Pain : Where do you feel pain? (e.g., sharp pain in the head for headache, ache in the legs after running)

  ✓ Fullness : Where do you feel fullness? (e.g., bloated stomach after a meal)

◉ Drawing and Writing
   ✓ Have the children draw or write about the sensations in the corresponding areas on their body map. They can use symbols, words, or shapes to depict their sensations.
   ✓ Example: Draw a red circle in the stomach area for hunger or blue drops near the throat for thirst.

Discussion

✓ Ask children to explain their body map, discussing where and how they feel different sensations.
✓ Encourage them to talk about any patterns they notice and how these sensations help them understand their body's needs.
✓ If in a Group - Comparing Maps:
   • Allow the children to compare their body maps with others.
   • Discuss similarities and differences in how they experience sensations. Questions to consider:
   • Did anyone feel hunger or thirst in the same place?
   • How do our bodies show us whether we are happy or tired?
   • Are there any surprising sensations that others felt differently?

OPTIONS : Provide stickers or other decorative items for children to personalize their body maps further. Use notebooks for children to write additional reflections or stories about their body sensations.

Benefits

✓ Interoceptive Awareness : Helps children understand and recognize their body's signals.
✓ Self-Expression : Encourages creative expression of internal experiences.
✓ Empathy and Understanding : Fosters discussions that highlight individual differences and commonalities in bodily sensations.
✓ Artistic Skills : Develops fine motor skills and creativity.

Conclusion : The Body Mapping Voyage is a powerful activity that combines art and introspection to help children visualize and understand their body sensations. By creating and discussing their body maps, children can develop a deeper awareness of their interoceptive signals, enhancing their ability to respond to their body's needs.

Cozy Corner Creation: Craft Your Personal Sanctuary

Overview

The Cozy Corner Creation activity guides children through the process of designing and setting up their own safe and calming space. This activity promotes emotional regulation and self-awareness by encouraging children to create a personalized area where they can relax and manage their emotions.

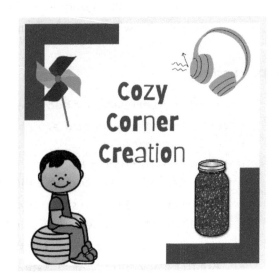

Goals

✓ Encourage self-awareness and emotional regulation.

✓ Foster creativity and a sense of ownership over personal space.

✓ Provide a tangible tool for managing stress and emotions.

Materials Needed

✓ Comfortable Seating: Cushions, bean bags, or a small chair.

✓ Soft Textiles: Blankets (soft or weighted), soft rugs, weighted or plush toys.

✓ Lighting: Soft lighting options such as fairy lights, a small lamp, or a night light.

✓ Decorative Items: Posters, pictures, or drawings that the child finds comforting or inspiring.

✓ Calming Tools: Items like stress balls, fidget toys, or sensory bottles.

✓ Aroma Therapy: Safe options like lavender sachets or essential oil diffusers.

✓ Quiet Activities: Books, coloring books, journals, or puzzles.

✓ Craft Supplies: Markers, crayons, paper, stickers, and other items for personalizing the space.

✓ Music: Any type of soft music that is preferred by the child.

✓ Sensory Bins: Containers filled with rice, beans, sand, or water beads for tactile exploration.

✓ Nature Elements: Smooth stones, pinecones, seashells, or small plants for a natural touch.

✓ Interactive Wall: Chalkboard, whiteboard, or felt board with various pieces to move and arrange.

✓ Bubble Tubes or Aquariums: For visual and auditory calming effects.

✓ Sound Machine: Offering a variety of soothing sounds like rain, ocean waves, or white noise.

✓ Tactile Wall Panels: Different textures like sandpaper, velvet, or faux fur for hands-on exploration.

✓ Visual Timers: Sand timers or liquid motion timers to help with time management and focus.

✓ Colorful Scarves or Ribbons: For sensory movement and visual stimulation.

- ✓ Rocking or Swivel Chair: To provide gentle motion.
- ✓ Activity Board: Featuring locks, latches, buttons, and zippers to engage fine motor skills.
- ✓ Therapy Putty or Playdough: For squeezing and shaping to relieve stress.
- ✓ Projection Night Light: That casts soothing images or patterns on the ceiling.
- ✓ Noise-Canceling Headphones: For blocking out overwhelming sounds.
- ✓ Magnetic Tiles or Blocks: For quiet, creative play and building.

Instructions

- ✓ Introduction
- ✓ Explain the purpose of a cozy corner: a place where children can go to feel calm, safe, and relaxed.
- ✓ Discuss how having a special area can help them manage their emotions and stress.

Choosing the Space

Help the child select a suitable location in their home. It could be a corner of their bedroom, a section of the living room, or even a small nook under a table. Ensure the space is quiet, private, and free from distractions.

Planning the Space

Talk about what makes the child feel calm and safe. This could include favorite colors, textures, and items. Make a list of items they would like to include in their calming space.

Gathering Materials

Collect the materials needed to set up the space. Involve the child in choosing and gathering items to give them a sense of ownership. Consider creating some DIY items, such as homemade stress balls, sensory bottles, or personalized art.

Setting Up the Space

- ✓ Start with the basics : Arrange comfortable seating and soft textiles.
- ✓ Add lighting : Use fairy lights or a small lamp to create a soothing ambiance.
- ✓ Incorporate calming tools : Place stress balls, fidget toys, or sensory bottles within easy reach.
- ✓ Add decorative items : Hang posters, pictures, or drawings that the child finds comforting or inspiring.
- ✓ Include quiet activities : Stock the space with books, coloring books, journals, or puzzles.

Personalizing the Space

- ✓ Allow the child to decorate the space with their artwork, stickers, or other craft items.
- ✓ Encourage them to create a name for their space, such as "Calm Corner" or "Peace Place."

Using the Space

Discuss when and how to use the calming space. Emphasize that it is a place to go when they need to relax, reflect, or manage their emotions. Practice using the space together. Model going to the space to take deep breaths or read a book.

Reflecting and Adjusting

After using the space for a while, ask the child how they feel about it. Make any necessary adjustments to improve comfort and effectiveness.

Benefits

✓ Emotional Regulation : Provides a designated area for children to manage their emotions.

✓ Creativity and Ownership : Encourages children to take ownership of their space and express their creativity.

✓ Stress Management : Offers tools and techniques to help children relax and de-stress.

Conclusion : Creating a cozy corner is a powerful tool for children to manage their emotions and find peace. By involving them in the setup and personalization of the space, you empower them to take control of their emotional well being.

Emotions Odyssey Activity

Overview

The Emotions Odyssey Activity is a dynamic and interactive adventure where children explore and act out various emotions through a series of imaginative challenges and games. This activity helps children understand and express their emotions in creative ways, promoting emotional literacy, empathy, and social skills.

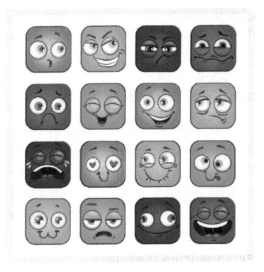

Goals

✓ Enhance emotional literacy by identifying and expressing various emotions.

✓ Develop empathy and understanding of others' emotions.

✓ Foster creativity, imagination, and dramatic skills.

✓ Improve communication skills and emotional regulation.

Materials Needed

✓ Emotion Cards : Cards with pictures and descriptions of different emotions. Cards are available in the resources section in the back of this book. It is always best to have actual photos of children acting out the emotions instead of cartoons or graphics.

✓ Emotion Odyssey Map : A map outlining different stations or checkpoints with various emotion-related challenges.

✓ Props and Costumes : Simple items like hats, scarves, masks, or toys to help children get into character.

✓ Activity Supplies : Depending on the tasks, you may need markers, paper, props, or other craft supplies.

Instructions

✓ Introduction : Explain the concept of the Emotions Odyssey and its purpose: to explore and understand different emotions through a series of fun and engaging challenges.

✓ Discuss the importance of recognizing and expressing emotions in a healthy way.

✓ Creating the Emotion Odyssey Map:

- Design a map with different stations or checkpoints, each representing a specific emotion. This map can be the same as in the Emotion Quest activity (in chapter 3) or can be different since the activities completed in this activity are different. For example:

- Station 1: Happiness

- Station 2: Sadness

- Station 3: Anger

- Station 4: Fear

- Station 5: Surprise

- Station 6: Disgust

- Station 7: Love

- Station 8: Calm

- Arrange the stations around the room, playground, or an outdoor area.

✓ Setting Up Stations:

- At each station, set up a unique activity that helps children explore the corresponding emotion. Examples include:

- Happiness Station: Dance party with happy music or drawing things that make them happy.

- Sadness Station: Storytime with a book about feeling sad, or a quiet space for reflection and drawing.

✓ Explaining the Odyssey :

- Give each child or group a copy of the Emotion Odyssey Map.

- Explain that they will visit each station, complete the activity, and collect a sticker or token for each completed task.

✓ Starting the Odyssey :

Allow the children to start the odyssey, moving from one station to another at their own pace. Encourage them to fully engage with each activity and express the designated emotion.

Discussion

✓ After completing the odyssey, gather the children for a group discussion.

✓ Ask them to share their favorite station and what they learned about their emotions.

✓ Discuss how understanding and expressing emotions can help them in everyday situations.

Conclusion : The Emotions Odyssey Activity is a fun and engaging way for children to explore their emotions through a variety of creative challenges. By participating in different activities and expressing their emotions, children can develop a deeper understanding of their feelings and learn healthy ways to express and manage them.

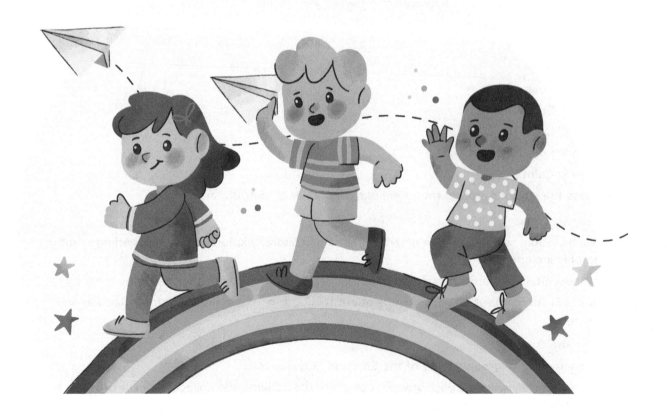

CHAPTER - 2

Decode Your Body's Messages
Sensory Sleuths

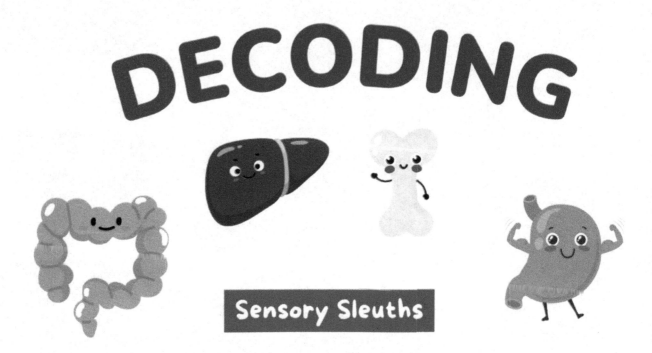

In this chapter, kids will become a sensory sleuths, decoding the messages their bodies send them every day. From hunger pangs to racing hearts, kids will learn to tune into their body's signals and understand what they mean. Interoception relies on a network of sensory receptors inside of every organ in the body. They detect internal changes, such as hunger, thirst, or pain. These signals are then relayed to the brainstem and thalamus before reaching the insular cortex for processing. Through engaging activities and hands-on experiments, kids will sharpen their senses and become experts at listening to what their bodies are telling them.

Sensory Scavenger Expedition

Overview : The Sensation Quest is an interactive and educational activity where children embark on a journey to match various sensations to the corresponding body parts. This activity helps enhance interoceptive awareness by teaching children to recognize where they feel different sensations in their bodies.

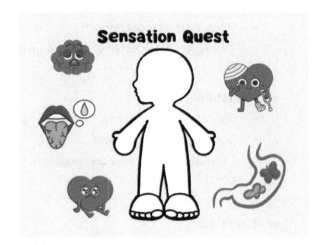

*Always give kids the opportunity to name their own body sensations. They may have creative and unique ways to describe what and where they feel

Goals

✓ Improve interoceptive awareness by linking sensations to body parts.

✓ Develop cognitive skills such as memory and matching.

✓ Encourage discussions about body awareness and sensations.

✓ Provide a fun and engaging way to learn about the body's signals.

Materials Needed

✓ Matching Cards : Sets of cards with images or descriptions of sensations (e.g., hunger, fast heartbeat) and body parts (e.g., stomach, heart). Cards for activity can be found in the resources section at the back of this book.

✓ Large Poster or Board : To display the body parts.

✓ Velcro Dots or Magnets : For attaching cards to the poster or board.

✓ Timer (Optional) : To make the game more exciting by adding a time element.

Instructions

✓ Introduction : Explain the purpose of the game: to match different sensations to the correct body parts. Discuss the importance of understanding where we feel different sensations in our bodies.

✓ Preparing the Game : Create or print matching cards. For each sensation, create a card with an image or description of the sensation and a separate card with the corresponding body part.

✓ Examples of sensations and body parts: Detailed Examples of Sensations

  ◉ **Hunger**
  - Description : Feeling of emptiness, rumbling, or gnawing in the stomach.
  - Body Part : Stomach
  - Example : When you have not eaten for several hours, you might feel a growling sensation in your stomach.

- ☑ **Thirst**
  - • Description : Dryness in the mouth or throat, desire to drink liquids.
  - • Body Part : Throat/Mouth
  - • Example : After playing outside on a hot day, you might feel a dry, scratchy throat.

- ☑ **Heartbeat**
  - • Description : Rhythmic or pounding heartbeat, often felt in the chest.
  - • Body Part : Heart/Chest
  - • Example : When you are excited or after running, you might feel your heart beating fast in your chest.

- ☑ **Tiredness**
  - • Description : Heavy eyelids, yawning, overall fatigue.
  - • Body Part : Entire Body/Eyes
  - • Example : After a long day at school, you might feel a heaviness in your eyes and a need to lie down.

- ☑ **Butterflies in the Stomach**
  - • Description : Fluttery feeling in the stomach, often due to nervousness or excitement.
  - • Body Part : Stomach
  - • Example : Before a big performance or test, you might feel a fluttery sensation in your stomach.

- ☑ **Shivers**
  - • Description : Trembling or shivering sensation, often due to cold or fear.
  - • Body Part : Skin and muscles
  - • Example : When you are cold or scared, you might feel shivers run down your spine or across your skin.

- ☑ **Warm Feeling**
  - • Description : A comforting or soothing warmth in the chest or body.
  - • Body Part : Chest
  - • Example : When you are happy or comforted, you might feel a warm sensation in your chest.

- ☑ **Muscle Soreness**
  - • Description : Aching or stiffness in muscles, often after physical activity.
  - • Body Part : Muscles
  - • Example : After playing sports or exercising, you might feel soreness in your legs or arms.

Headache

- Description : Pain or pressure in the head.
- Body Part : Head
- Example : If you are dehydrated or tired, you might feel a throbbing pain in your head.

Goosebumps

- Description : Tiny bumps on the skin, often caused by cold or strong emotions.
- Body Part : Skin
- Example : When you are cold or feel a strong emotion like excitement or fear, you might notice goosebumps on your arms.

Setting Up the Game

✓ Large Poster or Board : Draw or attach images of the body parts (stomach, throat, heart, etc.) in the appropriate locations on the poster or board.

✓ Playing the Game :

- Explaining the Game: Show the children the matching cards and explain how each card has either a sensation or a body part.
- Demonstrate how to match a sensation card to the corresponding body part card using an example.
- Divide the children into small groups or pairs.
- Give each group a set of matching cards.
- Allow the children to take turns picking a sensation card and matching it to the correct body part card on the poster or board.
- Use Velcro dots or magnets to attach the cards to the poster or board.
- Adding Excitement (Optional): Introduce a timer to add a competitive element. Set a time limit for each round and see which group can correctly match the most cards within the time.

Reflecting and Discussing

✓ After the game, gather the children to discuss what they learned.

✓ Ask questions such as:

✓ Which sensations were easy to match? Which were more difficult?

✓ How do you know where you feel different sensations in your body?

✓ Can you think of other sensations and where you feel them?

Adapting the Game

✓ For younger children, use simpler sensations and larger, more descriptive cards. Allow them to use their own words to describe what they feel.

✓ For older children, introduce more complex sensations and add descriptions to challenge their understanding.

Benefits

✓ Interoceptive Awareness : Helps children understand and recognize their body's signals.

✓ Cognitive Skills : Enhances memory, matching, and problem-solving abilities.

✓ Social Interaction : Encourages teamwork and discussion.

✓ Fun and Engagement : Provides a playful and educational experience.

Conclusion : The Sensation Quest: Match the Feeling to Your Body is a fun and educational activity that helps children develop a deeper understanding of their body's signals. By matching sensations to the correct body parts, children can improve their interoceptive awareness, cognitive skills, and emotional understanding.

Interoception Explorers: Discover Your Inner Signals Through Mindfulness

Explanation : Mindfulness is the practice of paying attention to the present moment with openness, curiosity, and without judgment. It helps children become more aware of their thoughts, feelings, and bodily sensations, enhancing their interoceptive abilities. Mindfulness can reduce stress, improve concentration, and promote emotional regulation. In this chapter, we will explore the science behind mindfulness and provide thrilling activities to help children practice mindfulness in fun and engaging ways.

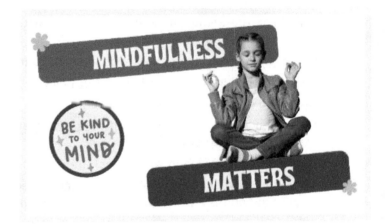

Why Mindfulness is Important:

✓ Increases Awareness : Mindfulness helps children become more aware of their internal states, such as hunger, thirst, and emotions. This awareness is crucial for developing strong interoceptive skills.

✓ Reduces Stress : Mindfulness practices can reduce anxiety and stress by calming the mind and body. It helps children cope with challenges and manage their emotions more effectively.

✓ Improves Focus : Regular mindfulness practice can enhance concentration and attention, making it easier for children to focus on tasks and learn new information.

✓ Promotes Emotional Regulation : Mindfulness helps children recognize and understand their emotions, leading to better self-control and emotional resilience.

✓ The Science of Mindfulness : Mindfulness impacts several areas of the brain and body:

✓ Prefrontal Cortex : This area of the brain is responsible for executive functions such as decision-making, attention, and self-control. Mindfulness practice strengthens this part of the brain, enhancing these skills.

- ✓ Amygdala : The amygdala is involved in processing emotions, particularly fear and stress. Mindfulness can reduce the activity of the amygdala, helping children feel calmer and less anxious.

- ✓ Hippocampus : This part of the brain is crucial for memory and learning. Mindfulness can increase the density of gray matter in the hippocampus, improving cognitive functions.

- ✓ Heart Rate and Breathing : Mindfulness practices, such as deep breathing, can lower heart rate and slow breathing, promoting a state of relaxation and reducing stress levels.

Overview

Interoception Explorers is an engaging and educational activity designed to help children understand interoception by participating in hands-on experiments that focus on recognizing and interpreting their body's internal signals. Through these experiments, children will learn how to identify sensations related to hunger, thirst, heart rate, and breathing.

Goals

- ✓ Enhance interoceptive awareness by focusing on internal body signals.
- ✓ Develop observational and analytical skills.
- ✓ Encourage discussions about how internal sensations relate to overall well-being.
- ✓ Provide a fun and interactive way to learn about interoception.

Materials Needed

- ✓ Stopwatch or Timer : To measure heart rate and breathing rate.
- ✓ Notebooks and Pencils : For recording observations.
- ✓ Water Bottles : To understand thirst signals.
- ✓ Snacks : To recognize hunger signals.
- ✓ Calming Music or Apps : For relaxation and mindfulness exercises.
- ✓ Exercise Space : An area to perform physical activities like jumping jacks or running in place.

Instructions

- ✓ Introduction: Explain the concept of interoception: the ability to sense internal body signals, such as hunger, thirst, heart rate, and breathing.
- ✓ Discuss how understanding these signals can help in recognizing and responding to the body's needs.

Sample Observation Table

CATEGORY	BEFORE	AFTER	EXPLANATION
Heart Rate	70 beats per minute	110 beats per minute	Your heartbeat was much faster after exercise, showing you were working hard.
Breathing Rate	15 breaths per minute	30 breaths per minute	You took more breaths after physical activity because your body needed more oxygen.
Thirst Awareness	Mouth felt fine, not dry	Mouth felt better after water	Your mouth felt dry before drinking but felt better after having some water.
Hunger Awareness	Stomach felt a bit empty	Stomach felt full after snack	Your tummy was growling a bit before eating but felt happy and full after having a snack.
Relaxation	Felt a little tense, shallow breaths	Felt calm and relaxed after exercise	You noticed tight shoulders and shallow breaths before but felt relaxed and breathed deeply after a mindfulness exercise.
Energy Levels	Felt tired and low on energy	Felt energetic and lively after nap	You were feeling tired before resting but felt full of energy after taking a nap.
Mood	Felt grumpy and irritable	Felt happy and cheerful after playtime	You were feeling grumpy before playing but felt happy and cheerful after playing with friends.
Concentration	Found it hard to focus	Focused better after a break	You had trouble focusing before taking a break but found it easier to concentrate afterward.

exPeRimenT 1 : HeaRT RaTe awaReneSS

Activity: Measuring Resting Heart Rate

- ✓ Have the children sit quietly and place their fingers on their wrists or necks to feel their pulse.

- ✓ Use a stopwatch to count the number of beats in 30 seconds, then double it to get the beats per minute (BPM). If children want to, they can simply count the number of beats in one minute. Double-check using a pulse oximeter if desired. We want kids to learn how to take their own heart rate as an objective way to understand their signs of stress for proactive relaxation activities before a possible meltdown.

- ✓ Record the resting heart rate in their notebooks.

Activity: Measuring Active Heart Rate

- ✓ Engage the children in a physical activity like jumping jacks or running in place for one minute. For children with decreased mobility, allow them to exercise their arms. Dancing to songs, such as the YMCA is a fun way to increase heart rate.

- ✓ Immediately after, have them measure their heart rate again using the same method.

- ✓ Record the active heart rate in their notebooks.

Discussion

Compare resting and active heart rates.

Discuss how physical activity affects heart rate and why it is important to listen to the body's signals.

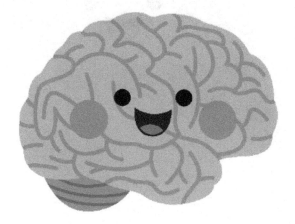

eXPeRimenT 2 : BReathing Rate awaReness

Activity: Measuring Resting Breathing Rate

✓ Have the children sit quietly and count their breaths (inhale and exhale) for one minute.

✓ Record the resting breathing rate in their notebooks.

Activity: Measuring Active Breathing Rate

✓ Engage the children in a physical activity for one minute.

✓ Immediately after, have them count their breaths for one minute.

✓ Record the active breathing rate in their notebooks.

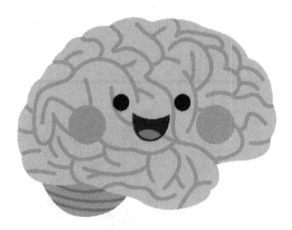

Discussion

Compare resting and active breathing rates.

Discuss how physical activity affects breathing and the importance of recognizing changes in breathing patterns.

eXPeRimenT 3 : HUNGeR anD ThiRST awaReneSS

Activity: Recognizing Thirst Signals

✓ Provide each child with a small water bottle.

✓ Have them take a sip of water and then wait for a few minutes.

✓ Ask them to note any changes in how they feel, particularly in their mouth and throat.

✓ During any activity, remind children to notice their own thirst and encourage drinking water.

✓ Record their observations in their notebooks.

Activity: Recognizing Hunger Signals

✓ Provide a small snack to each child.

✓ Before eating, ask them to note any hunger signals (e.g., stomach growling, feeling empty).

✓ After eating, ask them to note any changes in how they feel.

✓ Record their observations in their notebooks.

Discussion

Discuss the importance of listening to hunger and thirst signals.

Talk about how recognizing these signals can help in maintaining overall health and well-being.

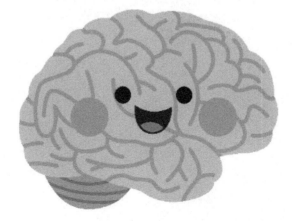

eXPeRimenT 4 : RelaXaTion anD minDfULNess

Activity: Guided Relaxation

✓ Play calming music or use a relaxation app.

✓ Guide the children through a simple mindfulness exercise, such as focusing on their breath or a body scan.

✓ After the exercise, ask them to note any sensations or changes in their body.

✓ Record their observations in their notebooks.

Discussion

Discuss the benefits of relaxation and mindfulness for recognizing and managing body signals.

Encourage the children to use these techniques when they feel stressed or overwhelmed.

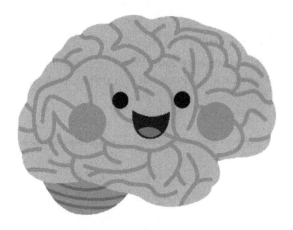

Benefits

✓ Interoceptive Awareness : Helps children understand and recognize their body's signals.

✓ Analytical Skills : Enhances observation, recording, and analysis of internal sensations.

✓ Emotional Regulation : Teaches techniques for managing stress and emotions.

✓ Engagement : Provides a hands-on, interactive learning experience.

Conclusion : Interoception Explorers: Discover Your Inner Signals is a comprehensive activity that combines physical exercises, mindfulness, and observational skills to help children understand and recognize their body's internal signals. By engaging in these experiments, children can develop a deeper awareness of interoception and learn valuable skills for maintaining their well-being.

Lotion Sensation

Activity : Lotion Sensation

Objective : To explore the sensation of touch by applying lotion and noticing how it feels on the skin.

Materials Needed

✓ Hand and foot lotion – always use unscented unless the child can choose the scent. The goal for this activity is to explore tactile sensations not scents.

✓ Towels or paper towels

✓ A comfortable space to sit

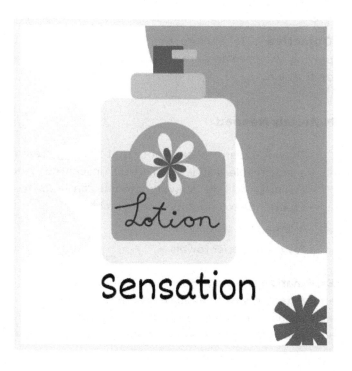

Explanation : Applying lotion to the hands and feet can help you become more aware of the sensations on your skin. This activity encourages mindfulness and helps you focus on the texture and temperature of the lotion as it is massaged into the skin.

Steps

◉ Get Comfortable : Find a comfortable place to sit where you can easily reach your hands and feet. Have the lotion and towels nearby.

◉ Introduction to the Activity : Explain that you will be exploring how lotion feels on your hands and feet. Encourage everyone to pay close attention to the sensations they experience.

- ☑ Apply Lotion to Hands :
  - Squeeze a small amount of lotion onto your hands. Rub your hands together, focusing on how the lotion feels as it spreads across your skin.
  - Notice the texture, temperature, and any changes in how your skin feels.
- ☑ Apply Lotion to Feet : Apply a small amount of lotion to your feet. Massage the lotion into your feet, paying attention to the sensations in your toes, heels, and soles.
- ☑ Discussion : After applying the lotion, discuss how your hands and feet feel. Use questions like:
  - "How did the lotion feel on your skin?"
  - "Did you notice any changes in temperature or texture?"
  - "How do your hands and feet feel now compared to before?"
  - "Did the lotion make your skin feel softer or smoother?"
  - "How did it feel to massage the lotion into your skin?"
  - "What was your favorite part of this activity?"
  - "Would you like to do this activity again? Why or why not?"

Shaving Cream Sensation

Objective : To explore the sensation of touch by playing with shaving cream and noticing how it feels on the skin.

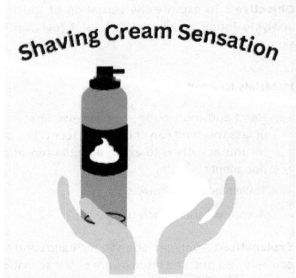

Materials Needed

- ✓ Shaving cream – Please note that shaving cream has a scent unless it is marked as unscented. Adding essential oils to shaving cream can add to the experience to engage sense of smell.
- ✓ A large tray or mat
- ✓ Towels or paper towels

Explanation : Playing with shaving cream is a fun and engaging way to explore different textures and sensations. This activity encourages sensory play and helps you become more aware of how your skin responds to touch.

Steps

- ☑ Set Up the Space : Lay down a large tray or mat to contain the shaving cream. Have towels or paper towels nearby for easy cleanup.
- ☑ Introduction to the Activity : Explain that you will be playing with shaving cream to explore how it feels on your hands and feet. Encourage everyone to focus on the sensations they experience.

- ☑ Apply Shaving Cream to Hands :
  - • Squeeze a generous amount of shaving cream onto the tray. Dip your hands into the shaving cream and rub them together, noticing the texture and temperature.
  - • Explore different ways to play with the shaving cream, such as squeezing, spreading, and piling it up.
- ☑ Apply Shaving Cream to Feet :
  - • Squeeze more shaving cream onto the tray. Dip your feet into the shaving cream and move them around, noticing how it feels between your toes and on your soles.
  - • Try making footprints or drawing patterns with your toes.
- ☑ Discussion : After playing with the shaving cream, discuss how your hands and feet feel. Use questions like:
  - • "How did the shaving cream feel on your skin?"
  - • "Did you notice any changes in temperature or texture?"
  - • "How do your hands and feet feel now compared to before?"
  - • "Did you enjoy the sensation of the shaving cream?"
  - • "What shapes or patterns did you create with the shaving cream?"
  - • "How did the shaving cream feel between your toes?"
  - • "Did you prefer using your hands or feet with the shaving cream?"
  - • "Would you like to try this activity with other materials? If so, what materials?"

Breezy Bliss

Activity : Feeling the Air

Objective : To explore the sensation of touch by feeling the air from a fan blowing on the skin.

Materials Needed

- ✓ A small fan
- ✓ A comfortable space to sit
- ✓ Towels or blankets (optional, for warmth)

Explanation : Feeling the air from a fan on your skin is a simple yet effective way to explore temperature and touch. This activity helps you become more aware of how your skin responds to changes in the environment.

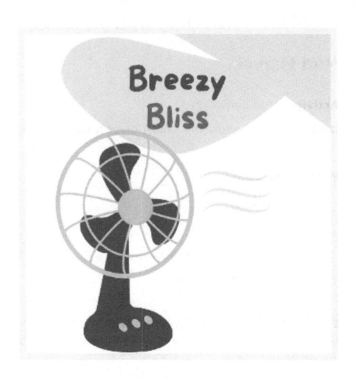

Steps

- ☑ Set Up the Space : Find a comfortable place to sit where you can easily feel the air from the fan. Place the fan nearby and have towels or blankets available if needed.

- ☑ Introduction to the Activity : Explain that you will be exploring how the air from the fan feels on your hands and feet. Encourage everyone to focus on the sensations they experience.

- ☑ Feel the Air on Your Hands :
  - Turn on the fan and hold your hands in front of it. Move your hands closer and further away from the fan to feel the difference in air intensity.
  - Notice the temperature and any changes in sensation as the air blows on your skin.

- ☑ Feel the Air on Your Feet :
  - Place your feet in front of the fan and move them closer and further away to feel the difference in air intensity.
  - Notice how the air feels on different parts of your feet, such as your toes, heels, and soles.

- ☑ Discussion : After feeling the air, discuss how your hands and feet feel. Use questions like:
  - "How did the air feel on your skin?"
  - "Did you notice any changes in temperature or intensity?"
  - "How do your hands and feet feel now compared to before?"
  - "Did the air from the fan make you feel cooler?"
  - "How did it feel when you moved closer to or further from the fan?"
  - "Did you prefer the sensation of air on your hands or feet?"
  - "How did the air feel on different parts of your feet?"
  - "Would you like to try this activity with a warm or cool breeze?"

Mud Marvel

Activity : Mud Sensation

Objective : To explore the sensation of touch by making and playing with mud.

Materials Needed

- ✓ Soil or dirt
- ✓ Water
- ✓ Large container or outdoor area
- ✓ Towels or paper towels

Explanation : Making and playing with mud is a fun way to explore different textures and sensations. This activity encourages sensory play and helps you become more aware of how your skin responds to different materials.

Steps

- ☑ Set Up the Space : Find a suitable outdoor area or use a large container to contain the mud. Have towels or paper towels nearby for easy cleanup.

- ☑ Introduction to the Activity : Explain that you will be making and playing with mud to explore how it feels on your hands and feet. Encourage everyone to focus on the sensations they experience.

- ☑ Make the Mud : Mix soil or dirt with water in the container or outdoor area until it reaches a mud-like consistency. Adjust the amount of water as needed to achieve the desired texture.

- ☑ Play with the Mud :

  - Dip your hands into the mud and rub them together, noticing the texture and temperature.

  - Explore different ways to play with the mud, such as squeezing, spreading, and piling it up.

  - Dip your feet into the mud and move them around, noticing how it feels between your toes and on your soles.

- ☑ Discussion : After playing with the mud, discuss how your hands and feet feel. Use questions like:

  - "How did the mud feel on your skin?"

  - "Did you notice any changes in temperature or texture?"

  - "How do your hands and feet feel now compared to before?"

  - "Did you enjoy playing with the mud?"

  - "What shapes or structures did you create with the mud?"

  - "How did the mud feel between your toes?"

  - "Did you prefer using your hands or feet with the mud?"

  - "Would you like to try this activity with other natural materials? If so, what materials?"

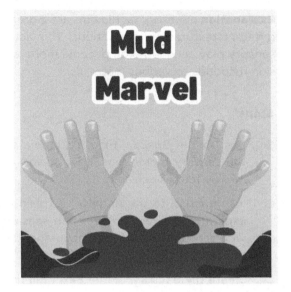

Tactile Treasure

Activity : Sensory Tactile Bins

Objective : To explore the sensation of touch by creating and playing with sensory tactile bins filled with various items.

Materials Needed

- ✓ Large bins or containers
- ✓ A variety of sensory items (at least 50 different items, see list below)
- ✓ Towels or paper towels

Explanation : Sensory tactile bins are a great way to explore different textures and sensations. This activity encourages sensory play and helps you become more aware of how your skin responds to various materials.

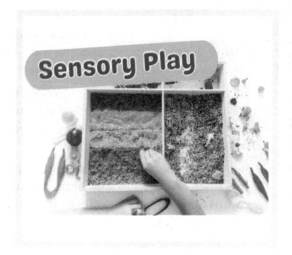

Steps

- ✔ Set Up the Space : Find a suitable space to set up the sensory tactile bins. Have towels or paper towels nearby for easy cleanup.

- ✔ Introduction to the Activity : Explain that you will be exploring different textures and sensations by playing with sensory tactile bins. Encourage everyone to focus on the sensations they experience.

- ✔ Create the Sensory Tactile Bins : Fill the bins or containers with a variety of sensory items. You can use one item per bin or mix several items together. Here are some ideas:

1.	Rice	18.	Shells	35.	Small plastic animals
2.	Beans	19.	Sponges	36.	Small plastic cars
3.	Sand	20.	Pipe cleaners	37.	Small plastic balls
4	Water beads	21.	Glitter	38.	Yarn
5.	Pom-poms	22.	Jingle bells	39.	Silk flowers
6.	Cotton balls	23.	Craft foam pieces	40.	Rice noodles
7.	Feathers	24.	Small toys	41.	Cooked spaghetti
8.	Buttons	25.	Bubble wrap	42.	Dried lentils
9.	Marbles	26.	Soft fabric pieces	43.	Small foam balls
10.	Dried pasta	27.	Dried leaves	44.	Small rubber balls
11.	Shredded paper	28.	Scented sachets	45.	Small wooden blocks
12.	Beads	29.	Ice cubes	46.	Paper confetti
13.	Sequins	30.	Warm water	47.	Sawdust
14.	Play dough	31.	Cool water	48.	Soil
15.	Flour	32.	Grass clippings	49.	Soft clay
16.	Cornstarch	33.	Pinecones	50.	Kinetic sand
17.	Small rocks	34.	Pine needles		

- ✔ Explore the Sensory Bins :
  - Dip your hands into the bins and explore the different textures. Move your hands around, squeeze, and feel the items.
  - Try using your feet to explore the bins, if appropriate.

- ✔ Discussion : After exploring the sensory bins, discuss how your hands and feet feel. Use questions like:
  - "Which items felt the most interesting?"
  - "Did you notice any changes in temperature or texture?"
  - "How do your hands and feet feel now compared to before?"

- "Which items did you enjoy touching the most?"

- "Did any items surprise you with how they felt?"

- "How did it feel to use your hands versus your feet?"

- "Did any items remind you of other experiences or sensations?"

- "Would you like to create your own sensory bin with your favorite items?"

Heartbeat Explorers: Build Your Own Stethoscope

Overview : Heartbeat Explorers is a creative and educational activity that guides children through the process of making a simple stethoscope. By constructing and using their own stethoscope, children can explore the sounds of their heartbeat and other body sounds, enhancing their understanding of interoception and the human body.

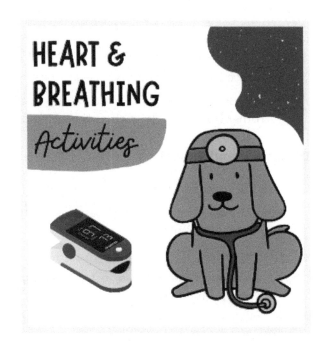

Goals

✓ Introduce basic concepts of how a stethoscope works.

✓ Enhance understanding of internal body sounds.

✓ Develop fine motor skills and problem-solving abilities.

✓ Encourage curiosity about the human body and healthcare tools.

Materials Needed

✓ Funnel : One small and one larger funnel (easily available at hardware stores or kitchen supply stores).

✓ Plastic Tubing : Approximately 2-3 feet of flexible plastic tubing (can be found in hardware stores).

✓ Tape : Strong adhesive tape or duct tape.

✓ Scissors : For cutting the tubing.

✓ Optional : Stethoscope ear tips (can be purchased online or at medical supply stores for added comfort).

Instructions

✓ Introduction : Explain what a stethoscope is and how doctors and nurses use it to listen to internal body sounds, such as the heartbeat and breathing.

✓ Discuss the importance of these sounds in monitoring health.

✓ Preparing the Materials:

- Gather all the materials needed for the stethoscope.

✓ - Cut the plastic tubing to the desired length (about 2-3 feet).

✓ Assembling the Stethoscope :

- Step 1 : Attach the larger funnel to one end of the plastic tubing. This will be the part placed against the body to capture sounds.
- Step 2 : Attach the smaller funnel to the other end of the plastic tubing. This will act as the part that amplifies the sound when placed in the ears.
- Step 3 : Secure the funnels to the tubing with strong adhesive tape. Ensure that there are no gaps where air can escape, as this will affect the sound quality.

Optional : If using stethoscope ear tips, attach them to the end of the smaller funnel for a more comfortable fit.

✓ Using the Stethoscope :

- Have the children sit quietly and place the larger funnel against their chest, over the heart.
- Place the smaller funnel (or ear tips) in their ears.
- Encourage them to listen carefully to the sounds of their heartbeat. They can also try listening to other body sounds, such as breathing or stomach gurgles.

Discussion and Reflection

✓ Ask the children what they heard and how it felt to use their homemade stethoscope.

✓ Discuss how doctors use stethoscopes in their daily work and why listening to internal body sounds is important for health.

✓ Exploration :

- Encourage the children to try listening to other sounds, such as a friend's heartbeat or breathing (with permission).
- They can also experiment with different body parts to hear various internal sounds.

✓ Safety Precautions :

- Ensure the tubing and funnels are clean before use.
- Make sure the children do not push the smaller funnel or ear tips too deeply into their ears to avoid injury.

Benefits

✓ Understanding Health Tools : Helps children learn about medical devices and their uses.

✓ Interoceptive Awareness : Enhances their ability to recognize and interpret internal body sounds.

✓ Fine Motor Skills : Develops their ability to assemble and handle small parts.

✓ Curiosity and Exploration : Encourages a deeper interest in science and health.

Conclusion : The Heartbeat Explorers: Build Your Own Stethoscope activity is a fun and educational way for children to explore the sounds of their bodies. By constructing their own stethoscope, they gain hands-on experience with a common medical tool and develop a greater understanding of how their bodies work. This activity fosters curiosity, learning, and a deeper appreciation for healthcare practices.

Backbone Bonanza: Craft Your Own Spine and Feel Your Bones

Overview : Backbone Bonanza is a fun and engaging activity where children create a model of a spine and explore the structure and function of their own backbones. This activity promotes awareness of the skeletal system and teaches children about the importance of the spine in supporting and protecting the body.

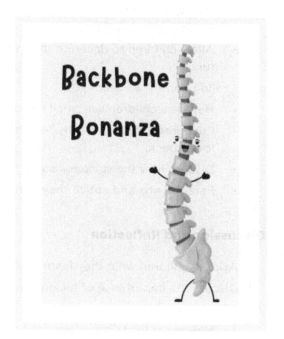

Goals

- ✓ Introduce the basic structure and function of the spine.
- ✓ Enhance understanding of the skeletal system.
  Develop fine motor skills and creativity.
- ✓ Encourage curiosity about the human body and its functions.

Materials Needed

- ✓ Pipe Cleaners : Approximately 12-15 pipe cleaners to represent the vertebrae.
- ✓ Beads : Assorted sizes and colors to represent the vertebrae and intervertebral discs.
- ✓ String or Yarn : To thread the beads and pipe cleaners.
- ✓ Scissors : For cutting string or yarn.
- ✓ Markers : For labeling or decorating the spine model.
- ✓ Small Mirrors : To help children see and feel their own spines.

Instructions

- ✓ Introduction: Explain the structure of the spine and its importance in supporting the body and protecting the spinal cord.
- ✓ Discuss the distinct parts of the spine: cervical, thoracic, lumbar, sacrum, and coccyx.
- ✓ Creating the Spine Model :
  - • Step 1: Cut a piece of string or yarn about 2 feet long.
  - • Step 2: Start by threading a larger bead (representing the cervical vertebrae) onto the string. Follow with a smaller bead (representing the intervertebral disc).
  - • Step 3: Alternate between larger beads (vertebrae) and smaller beads (discs) until you have a string of beads representing the entire spine.
  - • Step 4: To make the spine more realistic, use pipe cleaners to add "ribs" to the thoracic vertebrae section. Bend the pipe cleaners and twist them around the string between the beads.
  - • Step 5: Once all beads are threaded, tie a knot at each end of the string to keep the beads in place.

✓ Decorating and Labeling :
  - Use markers to label the different sections of the spine on the beads (e.g., C1-C7 for cervical, T1-T12 for thoracic, L1-L5 for lumbar).
  - Allow children to decorate their spine models with colors and patterns to make it more personal and fun.

✓ Feeling Their Own Spines :
  - Have the children use small mirrors to look at their own backs and locate their spines.
  - Encourage them to gently feel their vertebrae with their fingers, starting from the neck down to the lower back.
  - Discuss how the spine feels and moves, emphasizing its flexibility and strength.
  - Feel the ribs and notice their connections to make a safe place for the internal organs of the chest.

Discussion and Reflection

✓ Ask the children what they learned about the spine and its function.

✓ Discuss the importance of taking care of their spines through good posture, exercise, and safe practices.

✓ Extension Activity :
  - Movement Exploration: Have the children perform simple movements like bending forward, backward, and twisting to feel how their spines move.
  - Spine Health Tips: Share tips on maintaining a healthy spine, such as proper lifting techniques, regular physical activity, and good posture.

Spine Chart

✓ Neck (C1-C7) :
  - Top Neck Bone (C1) : Nods your head up and down, like saying "yes".
  - Second Neck Bone (C2) : Helps you turn your head side to side, like saying "no".
  - Neck Bones C3 to C7 : Support your neck and help you move your head in many ways.

✓ Upper Back (T1-T12) :
  - Upper Back Bones (T1 to T12) : Each bone is attached to a pair of ribs that help protect your heart and lungs.

✓ Lower Back (L1-L5) :
  - Lower Back Bones (L1 to L5) : These are the biggest and strongest bones in your back. They help you bend, twist, and carry the weight of your upper body.

✓ Hip Area (S1-S5) :
  - Hip Area Bones (S1 to S5) : These five bones are fused together to form the back part of your hips. They connect your spine to your hip bones.

✓ Tailbone (Co1-Co4) :
  - Tailbone Bones (Co1 to Co4) : Four small bones fused together to form your tailbone. They provide a place for muscles and ligaments in the pelvic area to attach and help support you when you sit.

Benefits

✓ Understanding the Skeletal System : Helps children learn about the spine's structure and function.

✓ Fine Motor Skills : Enhances coordination through threading and manipulating small objects.

✓ Creativity : Encourages artistic expression in decorating the spine model.

✓ Body Awareness : Increases awareness of their own bodies and promotes healthy habits.

Conclusion : Backbone Bonanza: Craft Your Own Spine and Feel Your Bones is a fun and educational way for children to learn about their spines. By creating a spine model and exploring their own spines, children gain a deeper understanding of the skeletal system and the importance of spine health. This activity fosters curiosity, learning, and a greater appreciation for their bodies.

Bone Discovery Adventure: Feel Your Bones

Overview : Bone Discovery Adventure is an interactive activity designed to help children explore and understand the bones in their bodies, including the elbows, chin, ribs, hands, and feet. By feeling and identifying these bones, children can enhance their body awareness and learn about the skeletal system in a fun and engaging way.

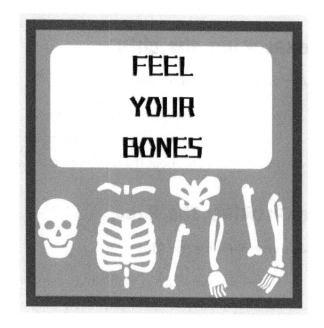

Goals

✓ Introduce children to the major bones in the body.

✓ Enhance body awareness and understanding of the skeletal system.

✓ Develop observational skills and tactile exploration.

✓ Encourage curiosity and learning about the human body.

Materials Needed

✓ Anatomy Book or Charts : Visual aids showing the skeletal system.

✓ Small Mirrors : For children to see and feel their own bones.

✓ Markers or Crayons : For drawing and labeling bones on paper.

✓ Paper and Pencils : For drawing and noting observations.

✓ Clay or Playdough : To model bones and joints.

Instructions

✓ Introduction :
  • Explain the purpose of the activity: to explore and feel the different bones in the body.
  • Discuss the importance of bones in providing structure, protection, and movement.

✓ Use the table on page 62 to guide you.

exploring The elbows

Activity: Feeling the Elbow Bones

✓ Have the children bend and straighten their elbows.

✓ Guide them to feel the bony protrusions on either side of their elbow (the ends of the humerus, radius, and ulna).

✓ Discussion : Explain how these bones come together to form the elbow joint and allow for bending and straightening of the arm.

exploring The chin

Activity: Feeling the Chin Bone

✓ Ask the children to gently touch their chin.

✓ Have them open and close their mouths to feel how the lower jaw (mandible) moves.

✓ Discussion: Talk about the mandible, its role in chewing and speaking, and how it connects to the skull.

exploring The Ribs

Activity: Feeling the Ribs

✓ Have the children place their hands on their chest and take a deep breath.

✓ Guide them to feel the ribcage expanding and contracting.

✓ Discussion: Explain the role of the ribs in protecting the lungs and heart, and how they are connected to the spine and sternum.

exploring The Hands

Activity: Feeling the Hand Bones

✓ Ask the children to wiggle their fingers and feel the bones in their hands.

✓ Have them touch the back of their hands to feel the metacarpal bones and the fingers to feel the phalanges.

✓ Discussion: Discuss the structure of the hand, the different types of bones (carpals, metacarpals, phalanges), and how they enable complex movements.

eXPLORiNG The FeeT

Activity: Feeling the Foot Bones

✓ Have the children remove their shoes and socks to feel the bones in their feet.

✓ Guide them to feel the heel (calcaneus), the arch (metatarsals), and the toes (phalanges).

✓ Discussion: Explain the structure of the foot, how it supports the body's weight, and allows for walking and running.

CReaTive eXPLORaTiON

Activity: Drawing and Labeling

✓ Provide paper and markers for the children to draw and label the bones they felt during the activity.

✓ Encourage them to create colorful and detailed diagrams.

Activity: Modeling Bones with Clay

✓ Use clay or playdough to model the different bones and joints explored in the activity.

✓ Have the children construct a simple skeleton or specific parts like the hand or foot.

Reflection and Discussion

✓ Ask the children to share their drawings and clay models.

✓ Discuss what they learned about their bones and how they help in everyday movements and activities.

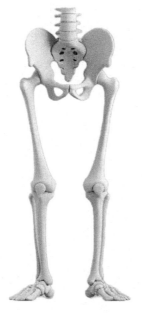

Sample Observation Table

BONE	LOCATION	FUNCTION
Humerus	Upper arm	Helps you move your arm
Radius/Ulna	Forearm	Lets you bend and twist your arm
Mandible	Lower jaw	Helps you chew food and talk
Ribs	Chest, around lungs and heart	Protects your lungs and heart
Metacarpals	Middle part of the hand	Makes up the palm of your hand
Phalanges	Fingers and toes	Helps you grip things and balance
Calcaneus	Heel bone	Supports you when you stand
Metatarsals	Middle part of the foot, forming arch	Gives your foot its shape and support
Femur	Thigh	Strong bone that helps you walk and run
Tibia	Shin	Helps you stand and walk
Fibula	Lower leg	Helps keep your ankle stable
Pelvis	Hips	Holds up your body and protects organs like your bladder
Clavicle	Collarbone	Connects your arm to your body, helping with shoulder movement
Scapula	Shoulder blade	Helps you move your shoulder and arm
Patella	Knee cap	Protects your knee
Vertebrae	Spine	Protects your spinal cord and helps you stand up straight
Cranium	Skull	Protects your brain
Sternum	Chest, center	Protects your heart and lungs

Benefits

✓ Understanding the Skeletal System : Helps children learn about the structure and function of different bones.

✓ Body Awareness : Increases awareness of their own bodies and promotes healthy habits.

✓ Fine Motor Skills : Enhances coordination through drawing and modeling.

✓ Creativity : Encourages artistic expression in drawing and modeling bones.

Conclusion : Bone Discovery Adventure: Feel Your Bones is a fun and educational way for children to learn about their bones. By exploring and identifying the bones in their elbows, chin, ribs, hands, and feet, children gain a deeper understanding of the skeletal system and the importance of bone health. This activity fosters curiosity, learning, and a greater appreciation for their bodies.

Muscle Magic: Exploring How Muscles Work

Overview : Muscle Magic is a hands-on activity designed to help children understand how muscles work. By engaging in a series of interactive exercises, including the Floating Arm activity, children can learn about muscle contraction, relaxation, and how muscles work in pairs to move the body.

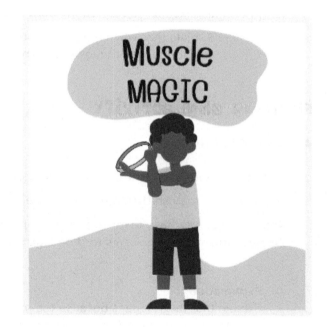

Goals

✓ Introduce the basic functions of muscles.

✓ Enhance understanding of muscle contraction and relaxation.

✓ Demonstrate how muscles work in pairs to create movement.

✓ Encourage physical activity and body awareness.

Materials Needed

✓ Elastic Bands : To simulate muscle contraction.

✓ Small Weights : For demonstrating muscle strength (optional).

✓ Paper and Markers : For drawing and labeling muscle groups.

✓ Mirrors : For observing muscle movement.

✓ Wall Space : For the Floating Arm activity.

Instructions

✓ Introduction to Muscles :

- Explain that muscles are tissues in the body that can contract and relax to create movement.

- Discuss how muscles work in pairs; when one muscle contracts, its partner muscle relaxes. For example, the biceps and triceps in the arm.

Activity: Muscle Contraction with Elastic Bands

✓ Step 1: Give each child an elastic band. Make sure the band is not too tight and can stretch easily.

✓ Step 2: Have the children hold the elastic band with both hands, about shoulder-width apart.

✓ Step 3: Instruct them to stretch the band by pulling their hands apart. Explain that this simulates muscle contraction, where the muscle fibers shorten and create tension.

✓ Step 4: Release the tension slowly to simulate muscle relaxation, where the muscle fibers lengthen and reduce tension.

✓ Step 5: Repeat this action several times, encouraging the children to observe how the band shortens and lengthens, just like muscles do during contraction and relaxation.

✓ Discussion: Explain that when muscles contract, they pull on the bones to create movement. When they relax, they allow the bones to move back to their resting positions.

FLOaTiNg aRM acTiViTY

Activity: Floating Arm

✓ Have the children stand next to a wall with one arm pressed against it.

✓ Instruct them to push their arm against the wall with moderate force for about 30 seconds.

✓ After 30 seconds, have them step away from the wall and let their arm relax.
Observe how their arm seems to "float" up involuntarily.

> **Explanation :**
> Explain that this happens because the muscles involved in pushing against the wall (the deltoid and other shoulder muscles) continue to contract even after stopping the push, causing the arm to lift.

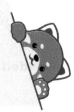

DeMONSTRaTiNg MUSCLe PaiRS

Activity: Biceps and Triceps

✓ Have children feel their biceps and triceps while bending and straightening their arms.

✓ Explain how the biceps contract to bend the arm and the triceps contract to straighten it.

✓ Activity: Drawing and Labeling Muscles

✓ Provide paper and markers for children to draw an arm and label the biceps and triceps.

✓ Encourage them to draw arrows showing how the muscles work in pairs.

MUSCLE STRENGTH DEMONSTRATION

Activity: Lifting Weights

✓ Use small weights or objects to demonstrate muscle strength.

✓ Have children lift weights and observe how their muscles contract.

Discussion

✓ Discuss how regular exercise can strengthen muscles and improve their function.
Reflection and Discussion:

✓ Ask the children to share their observations from the activities.

✓ Discuss the importance of muscles in everyday activities and how to keep muscles healthy through exercise and proper nutrition.

Benefits

✓ Understanding Muscle Function : Helps children learn about muscle contraction and relaxation.

✓ Body Awareness . Increases awareness of their own muscles and how they work.

✓ Physical Activity : Encourages physical movement and exercise.

✓ Creativity : Enhances understanding through drawing and labeling muscle groups.

Conclusion : Muscle Magic: Exploring How Muscles Work is a fun and educational activity that helps children learn about their muscles. Through interactive exercises and the Floating Arm activity, children gain a deeper understanding of muscle function and the importance of muscles in movement. This activity fosters curiosity, learning, and a greater appreciation for their bodies.

Sounds of Discovery: Exploring Hearing

Overview: Sounds of Discovery is an interactive activity designed to help children explore the sense of hearing. Through a series of engaging exercises, children will learn how their ears work, identify different sounds, and understand the importance of hearing in everyday

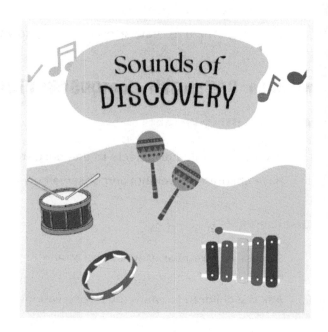

Goals

✓ Introduce the basic anatomy and function of the ear.

✓ Enhance understanding of how hearing works.

✓ Develop listening skills and sound recognition.

✓ Encourage curiosity about the sense of hearing.

Materials Needed

✓ Anatomy Book or Charts : Visual aids showing the structure of the ear.

✓ Sound Clips or Instruments : A variety of sounds or musical instruments

✓ Blindfolds : For sound identification games.

✓ Paper and Markers : For drawing and noting observations.

✓ Empty Containers : For creating DIY instruments.

✓ Materials for Instruments: Items like rice, beans, bells, rubber bands, etc.

✓ Balloons: To feel vibrations.

✓ Additional DIY Instrument Materials: Straws, bottle caps, cardboard tubes, plastic bottles, aluminum foil, etc.

Instructions

✓ Introduction to Hearing :

- Explain the structure of the ear and how it works, using anatomy books or charts.
- Discuss the three main parts of the ear: the outer ear, middle ear, and inner ear, and their roles in hearing.

Listening and identifying sounds

Activity: Sound Scavenger Hunt

- ✓ Play various sound clips or use musical instruments to create different sounds. Include sounds of nature.
- ✓ Ask the children to close their eyes or wear blindfolds and identify each sound.
- ✓ Discuss how they recognized each sound and what it reminds them of.

Activity: Sound Mapping

- ✓ Take the children outside or around the classroom.
- ✓ Have them sit quietly and listen to the sounds around them
- ✓ Ask them to draw a map of the area and mark where each sound is coming from (e.g., birds chirping, cars passing, people talking).

Making DIY instruments

Activity: Crafting Instruments

- ✓ Provide empty containers and various materials like rice, beans, bells, rubber bands, etc.
- ✓ Guide the children in making their own simple instruments, such as shakers, drums, or rubber band guitars.
- ✓ Encourage them to experiment with different materials to create unique sounds.

Ideas for DIY instruments

Activity: Crafting Instruments

- ✓ Shaker: Fill an empty container (like a plastic bottle or can) with rice, beans, or small beads. Seal it tightly and shake to produce sound.
- ✓ Drum : Use an empty container (like a coffee can) and stretch a piece of balloon or plastic wrap over the top. Secure it with a rubber band and tap to create a drum sound.
- ✓ Rubber Band Guitar : Stretch rubber bands of different thicknesses around an empty tissue box or a cardboard tube. Pluck the rubber bands to produce different pitches
- ✓ Kazoo : Use a cardboard tube (like a toilet paper roll) and cover one end with wax paper, securing it with a rubber band. Hum into the open end to create a buzzing sound.
- ✓ Pan Flute : Cut straws of different lengths and tape them together in a row. Blow across the tops to create different pitches.
- ✓ Bottle Cap Cymbals : Attach two bottle caps to each end of a string or rubber band. Clap the caps together to create a cymbal sound.

SOUND AND VIBRATION EXPERIMENT

Activity: Feeling Vibrations with Balloons

- ✓ Inflate balloons and have the children hold them.
- ✓ Play music or create sounds by talking near the balloon.
- ✓ Ask the children to feel the vibrations through the balloon.
- ✓ Explain how sound waves create vibrations that our ears detect as sound.

Alternative Activity: Rubber Band Vibration

- ✓ Stretch a rubber band around an empty container or box.
- ✓ Pluck the rubber band to create vibrations and sound.
- ✓ Have children observe how the sound changes with different tension levels and materials.
- ✓ Discuss how vibrations are an essential part of hearing.

EXPLORING HIGH AND LOW PITCHES

Activity: Pitch Comparison

- ✓ Play sounds of varying pitches, both high and low.
- ✓ Ask the children to identify if the sound is high-pitched or low-pitched.
- ✓ Discuss how different pitches are produced and why some sounds are higher or lower than others.

Reflection and Discussion

- ✓ Ask the children to share their favorite part of the activity and what they learned about hearing.
- ✓ Discuss the importance of protecting their ears and hearing health, such as avoiding loud noises and using ear protection.

Benefits

- ✓ Understanding Hearing: Helps children learn about the ear's structure and how hearing works.
- ✓ Listening Skills : Enhances their ability to recognize and differentiate sounds.
- ✓ Creativity : Encourages artistic expression through crafting instruments.
- ✓ Scientific Curiosity : Fosters an interest in science through hands-on experiments.

Conclusion : Sounds of Discovery: Exploring Hearing is a fun and educational activity that helps children learn about their sense of hearing. Through interactive exercises and creative projects, children gain a deeper understanding of how their ears work and the importance of hearing in their daily lives. This activity fosters curiosity, learning, and a greater appreciation for the sense of hearing.

Vision Exploration: Fun with Sight

Overview: Vision Exploration is an engaging activity designed to help children understand and appreciate their sense of sight. Through a series of fun and interactive exercises, children will learn how their eyes work, explore visual illusions, and understand the importance of vision in everyday life.

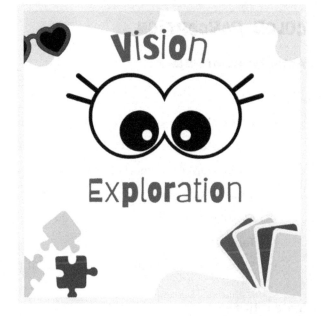

Goals

- ✓ Introduce the basic anatomy and function of the eye.
- ✓ Enhance understanding of how vision works.
- ✓ Develop observational skills and visual perception.
- ✓ Encourage curiosity about the sense of sight.

Materials Needed

- ✓ Anatomy Book or Charts: Visual aids showing the structure of the eye.
- ✓ Magnifying Glasses : For exploring objects up close.
- ✓ Color Filters or Glasses : To explore how colors are perceived.
- ✓ Optical Illusions : Printed examples of visual illusions.
- ✓ Paper and Markers : For drawing and noting observations.
- ✓ Mirrors: For exploring reflections.
- ✓ Objects for Observation: Leaves, insects, small toys, etc.
- ✓ Additional Visual Perception Game Materials: Items like patterned paper, puzzles, picture books, spot-the-difference images, and matching cards.

Instructions

- ✓ Introduction to Vision :
  - • Explain the structure of the eye and how it works, using anatomy books or charts.
  - • Discuss the main parts of the eye: the cornea, lens, retina, and optic nerve, and their roles in vision.

EXPLORING CLOSE-UP VISION

Activity: Magnifying Glass Exploration

✓ Provide magnifying glasses and a variety of small objects like leaves, insects, and toys.

✓ Encourage the children to observe the objects up close and note the details they can see with the magnifying glass.

✓ Discuss how the magnifying glass helps them see details that are not visible to the naked eye.

COLOR PERCEPTION

Activity: Color Filters

✓ Provide :

- Color filters or glasses in red, blue, green, and yellow
- Various colored objects (e.g., toys, paper, fabrics)
- White paper and markers or crayons
- Observation sheets for recording findings
- Flashlight or natural light source
- Tape
- Scissors (if color filters need to be cut to size)

Instructions

⦿ Introduction :

- Begin with a brief explanation of light and color. Explain that white light is made up of all the colors of the rainbow.
- Introduce the concept of color filters and how they work by allowing only certain colors of light to pass through.

⦿ Exploring with Color Filters :

- Distribute the color filters or glasses to the children.
- Have them take turns looking at different objects through each color filter. Encourage them to describe what they see.
- Provide observation sheets for children to record their observations. They should note the original color of the object and how it appears through each filter.

- **Hands-On Experiment :**
  - Set up a table with various colored objects and provide enough space for children to move around and observe.
  - Ask the children to choose one object at a time and look at it through each color filter. They should record their observations on the observation sheets.
  - Repeat the process with several objects of different colors.
- **Group Discussion :**
  - After everyone has had a chance to explore with the filters, gather the children for a group discussion.
  - Discuss their observations. Ask questions like:
    - How did the red object look through the blue filter?
    - Did any colors look the same through certain filters?
    - Were there any surprises in how colors changed?
- **Explanation and Learning :**
  - Explain why the colors changed when viewed through the filters. Discuss how each filter blocks certain wavelengths of light and only allows its own color to pass through.
  - Use a simple diagram to show how light passes through a filter and how the filter affects the colors we see.
- **Advanced Exploration :**
  - Introduce the concept of additive and subtractive color mixing. Use colored lights (flashlights with color filters) to demonstrate how combining different colors of light can create new colors.
  - For example, shine a red and green filtered flashlight on a white surface and observe the result.

Where to Purchase Colored Filters: Craft stores, school supply stores (Lakeshore or Discount School Supply), photography stores, Amazon

Additional Information about Color Filters:

- **How Color Filters Work:** Color filters are materials that selectively transmit light of certain colors. They block other wavelengths, allowing only their own color to pass through. For example, a red filter allows red light to pass through while blocking other colors.
- **Types of Color Filters :**
  - Absorptive Filters **:** Made from colored glass or plastic, these filters absorb specific wavelengths.
  - Dichroic Filters : Use coatings to reflect certain wavelengths and transmit others, often used in photography and stage lighting.
- **Applications of Color Filters :**
  - Photography and Filmmaking : To create different lighting effects and moods.
  - Theater Lighting : For colored lighting effects on stage.
  - Scientific Research : To isolate specific wavelengths for analysis.

OPTicaL iLLUSiONS

Activity: Exploring Optical Illusions

Download or print optical illusions, such as the famous "vase or two faces" illusion, the "impossible triangle," and "moving dots."

- ✓ Hermann Grid Illusion : Dark spots appear at the intersections of a white grid on a black background.
- ✓ Kanizsa Triangle : An illusionary white triangle appears due to the arrangement of three Pac-Man-like shapes.
- ✓ Café Wall Illusion : Straight lines appear wavy when a staggered grid of black and white tiles is viewed.
- ✓ Ponzo Illusion : Two identical horizontal lines appear different in length due to converging lines (like a railroad track).
- ✓ Müller-Lyer Illusion : Two identical lines appear different in length because of arrowheads at their ends .
- ✓ Ambiguous Cylinder Illusion : Cylinders appear circular or square depending on the viewpoint and reflection.
- ✓ Rotating Snakes : A static image with a pattern of circles appears to move and spin.
- ✓ Impossible Trident (Blivet) : A drawing that looks like it has three cylindrical prongs at one end and merges into two rectangular prongs at the other.
- ✓ Ebbinghaus Illusion : Two identical circles appear different in size due to the surrounding circles.
- ✓ Zöllner Illusion : Parallel lines appear to be angled due to the background of short lines crossing them.

Have the children observe each illusion and describe what they see. Discuss how optical illusions trick our eyes and brains, and why they occur.

ReFLeCTiON aND SYMMeTRY

Activity: Mirror Exploration

- ✓ Provide mirrors and have the children explore reflections by looking at themselves and objects in the mirror.
- ✓ Encourage them to create symmetrical drawings by folding paper in half and drawing one half of an image, then pressing the paper together to transfer the ink and create a symmetrical design.
- ✓ Discuss the concept of symmetry and how reflections work.

ViSUaL PeRCePTiON games

Activity: "I Spy" Game

- ✓ Play a game of "I Spy" where children take turns describing objects they see in the room or outdoors using descriptive words.
- ✓ Encourage them to use their observational skills to find objects that match the descriptions.

Activity: Shape and Color Hunt

✓ Give the children a list of shapes and colors to find around the room or outdoors.

✓ Have them check off each item as they find it, encouraging them to notice details in their environment.

Activity: Spot the Difference

✓ Provide images with slight differences and have the children identify the differences between them.

✓ Discuss how paying attention to detail helps improve their observational skills.

Activity: Picture Puzzles

✓ Use simple jigsaw puzzles or picture puzzles to help children recognize patterns and complete the images.

✓ Discuss how solving puzzles requires careful observation and problem-solving skills.

Activity: Matching Pairs

✓ Create matching cards with pictures, shapes, or colors. Have the children find and match the pairs.

✓ Discuss how recognizing similarities and differences is important for visual perception.

Activity: Hidden Pictures

✓ Provide books or printed images with hidden objects and have the children find the hidden items.

✓ Discuss how focusing and scanning help in locating hidden objects.

Reflection and Discussion

✓ Ask the children to share their favorite part of the activity and what they learned about vision.

✓ Discuss the importance of taking care of their eyes, such as eating healthy foods, wearing sunglasses, and taking breaks from screens.

Benefits

✓ Understanding Vision : Helps children learn about the eye's structure and how vision works.

✓ Observational Skills : Enhances their ability to notice details and describe what they see.

✓ Creativity : Encourages artistic expression through drawing and creating optical illusions.

✓ Scientific Curiosity : Fosters an interest in science through hands-on experiments and games.

Conclusion : Vision Exploration: Fun with Sight is a fun and educational activity that helps children learn about their sense of vision. Through interactive exercises and creative projects, children gain a deeper understanding of how their eyes work and the importance of vision in their daily lives. This activity fosters curiosity, learning, and a greater appreciation for the sense of sight.

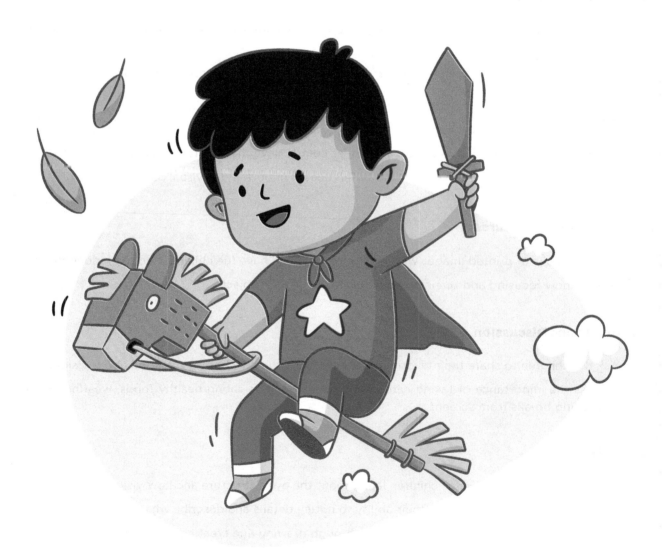

CHaPTeR - 3

eMOTioNS aND FeeLiNgS

Messages of the Heart

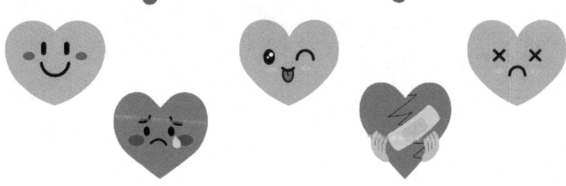

Understanding and naming emotions is a crucial part of interoception. Emotions are complex experiences that involve our bodies and minds. Our emotions depend on our past experiences. For example, a child may become upset at the sound of sirens or fire drills. Negative emotions can occur when kids are triggered by sensory experiences, and they remember a situation in which they were not comfortable. Sounds kids love such as the ice cream truck music or their caregiver's voice evoke positive emotions. In this way, they can affect how we think, feel, and behave. This chapter will explore the science of emotions, provide a list of common emotions and feelings words, and offer thrilling activities to help children identify and express their emotions effectively.

Why Understanding Emotions is Important

- Emotional Awareness : Recognizing and naming emotions helps children understand their internal experiences and how these emotions influence their thoughts and actions.

- Emotional Regulation : Being aware of emotions is the first step in learning how to manage them. Children can use this awareness to develop strategies for coping with difficult emotions.

- Social Skills : Understanding their own emotions helps children empathize with others and develop better communication and relationship skills.

- Mental Health : Awareness and expression of emotions contribute to overall mental well-being, reducing the risk of anxiety and depression.

The Science of Emotions : Emotions are responses to significant internal and external events. They involve:

- Physiological Responses : Changes in heart rate, breathing, and muscle tension, sweating, facial flushing, shaking, chills/goosebumps, crying.

- Expressive Behaviors : Facial expressions, body language, and tone of voice. This can be difficult for kids when first learning about interoception because they need to make connections between the sensations they feel and the associated emotions.

- Cognitive Processes : Thoughts and interpretations of the situation. Attention, decision-making, memory formation and retrieval, executive function.

Emotions are processed in different parts of the brain and body, involving a complex interaction between various systems:

- The Limbic System : Often referred to as the "emotional brain," the limbic system includes structures like the amygdala, hippocampus, and hypothalamus. It plays a key role in processing emotions, forming memories, and regulating autonomic responses.

  - Amygdala : The amygdala is crucial for processing emotions, especially those related to survival, such as fear and anger. It helps us recognize emotional stimuli and react quickly.

  - Hippocampus : This structure is essential for forming new memories and connecting emotions to these memories. It helps us remember emotional experiences and learn from them.

  - Hypothalamus : The hypothalamus links the nervous system to the endocrine system via the pituitary gland, helping regulate emotional responses through hormone release.

- Prefrontal Cortex : The prefrontal cortex is involved in higher-order functions such as decision-making, problem-solving, and regulating emotions. It helps us control impulsive reactions and engage in thoughtful responses.

  - Orbitofrontal Cortex : This area within the prefrontal cortex is important for evaluating emotional experiences and making decisions based on anticipated rewards and punishments.

  - Ventromedial Prefrontal Cortex : It plays a role in processing risk and fear, helping us navigate social interactions and make moral judgments.

- **Insula** : The insula is involved in interoceptive awareness, connecting physical sensations with emotional experiences. It helps us become aware of bodily states that accompany different emotions, such as the butterflies in our stomach when nervous or a pounding heart when excited.

- **Autonomic Nervous System (ANS)** : The ANS controls involuntary bodily functions and has two main branches:

  - **Sympathetic Nervous System** : Responsible for the "fight or flight" response, it prepares the body for action by increasing heart rate, dilating pupils, and releasing adrenaline.

  - **Parasympathetic Nervous System** : Promotes the "rest and digest" response, helping the body relax and recover by slowing the heart rate and increasing digestion.

- **Endocrine System** : Emotions are also influenced by hormones released by the endocrine system, such as cortisol (stress hormone), adrenaline (fight or flight response), and oxytocin (associated with bonding and trust).

Understanding the interplay between these systems helps us comprehend how emotions are generated and regulated. This knowledge can empower children to better understand their emotional experiences and develop effective strategies for managing them.

List of Emotions and Feelings Words

Charts :

Create visual charts to help children recognize and name their emotions. These charts can include facial expressions, body language cues, and descriptive words.

Emotions Faces Chart:

- **Description** : A chart with different faces showing various emotions. Each face is labeled with the corresponding emotion word. Emotions downloads are available in the resources section at the end of this book.

- **Purpose** : Help children match facial expressions with emotion words to improve recognition and naming skills.

Feelings Words Chart

- **Description** : A colorful chart with emotion words grouped by categories (e.g., happy, sad, angry). Each word is accompanied by a simple icon or illustration.

- **Purpose** : Expand children's emotional vocabulary and help them find the right words to describe their feelings. This can take lots of practice so be patient with kids as they learn.

Body Language and Emotions Chart:

- **Description** : A chart showing different body language cues associated with various emotions (e.g., crossed arms for anger, slumped shoulders for sadness).

✓ **Purpose :** Teach children how body language can express emotions and help them become more aware of their own and others' non-verbal signals.

Emotion Spectrum Paint Chips

Overview: To help children recognize and articulate their emotions and feelings through interoceptive awareness using a creative and engaging paint chip activity.

Materials Needed

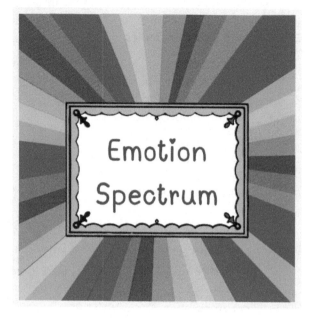

✓ Paint chips in various shades and colors (can be obtained from a hardware store)

✓ Binder ring

✓ Markers or pens

✓ Labels or small stickers

✓ A poster board or large sheet of paper

✓ Glue or tape

Instructions

✓ Introduction:

- Begin by explaining the concept of emotions and feelings, highlighting how they can vary in intensity and type.
- Introduce the idea of interoceptive awareness, explaining that it involves understanding the physical sensations inside our bodies that are linked to emotions (e.g., a racing heart when scared).

Optional Labels for Physical Sensations

✓ Happiness : Lightness in the chest, smiling, warmth in the body.

✓ Sadness : Heaviness in the chest, tearfulness, a sinking feeling in the stomach.

✓ Anger : Heat in the face, clenched fists, a fast heartbeat.

✓ Calmness : Steady breathing, relaxed muscles, a peaceful mind.

✓ Fear : Butterflies in the stomach, sweating, a racing heart.

✓ Excitement : Tingling in the body, increased energy, wide eyes.

✓ Love : Warmth in the heart, a sense of connection, smiling.

✓ Disgust : Nausea, wrinkling the nose, pulling back.

✓ Surprise : Raised eyebrows, widened eyes, a gasp.

✓ Contentment : A relaxed smile, steady breathing, a warm feeling in the chest.

✓ Confusion : Furrowed brows, scratching the head, a puzzled look.

✓ Frustration : Tension in the shoulders, a tight jaw, a feeling of being stuck.

Choosing Paint Chips

✓ Allow the children to choose paint chips that represent different emotions. For example, shades of blue for sadness, red for anger, yellow for happiness, green for calmness, etc.

✓ Encourage them to select a range of shades for each emotion to represent different intensities (e.g., light blue for mild sadness, dark blue for intense sadness).

Emotion and Color Examples

✓ Happiness :
  - Yellow (bright, cheerful)
  - Light Yellow (mild happiness)
  - Golden Yellow (intense joy)

✓ Sadness :
  - Blue (calm, melancholic)
  - Light Blue (mild sadness)
  - Navy Blue (deep sorrow)

✓ Anger :
  - Red (intense, fiery)
  - Light Red (mild irritation)
  - Dark Red (fury)

✓ Calmness .
  - Green (peaceful, serene)
  - Light Green (mild calmness)
  - Forest Green (deep relaxation)

✓ Fear :
  - Grey (uncertainty, apprehension)
  - Light Grey (mild anxiety)
  - Dark Grey (intense fear)

✓ Excitement :
  - Orange (energetic, enthusiastic)
  - Light Orange (mild excitement)
  - Deep Orange (bursting excitement)

✓ Love :
  - Pink (warm, affectionate)
  - Light Pink (gentle love)
  - Deep Pink (passionate love)

✓ Disgust :
  - Brown (rejection, aversion)
  - Light Brown (mild disgust)
  - Dark Brown (strong aversion)

✓ Surprise :
  - Purple (unexpected, astonished)
  - Light Purple (mild surprise)
  - Deep Purple (shock)

✓ Contentment :
  - Beige (satisfied, at ease)
  - Light Beige (mild contentment)
  - Tan (deep satisfaction)

✓ Confusion :
  - Teal (uncertainty, puzzlement)
  - Light Teal (mild confusion)
  - Dark Teal (deep puzzlement)

✓ Frustration :
  - Maroon (irritation, blocked)
  - Light Maroon (mild frustration)
  - Deep Maroon (intense frustration)

Labeling Emotions

✓ On each paint chip, have the children write the emotion it represents and add a brief description of the physical sensations associated with that emotion. For example, "Happy: Warm, light feeling in the chest."

✓ Use labels or stickers to help organize the paint chips by emotion category.

Creating the Emotion Spectrum

✓ Option 1 : Arrange the labeled paint chips on a poster board or large sheet of paper in a way that shows the spectrum of emotions and their intensities. Glue or tape the paint chips in place, creating a visual representation of the emotional spectrum.

✓ Option 2 : Use a hole puncher to create a hole in the top of each paint chip. Combine chips onto a binder ring. Allow children to take the ring and keep it with them. Encourage them to use the ring to help identify emotions as they occur to help with emotional awareness and to know when to implement calming strategies to prevent stress reactions.

Discussion

✓ Discuss with the children how different emotions feel in their bodies and how recognizing these feelings can help them understand and manage their emotions better.

✓ Encourage them to share their own experiences and physical sensations linked to various emotions.

Reflection

✓ Conclude the activity by reflecting on how the children can use this new awareness in their daily lives.

✓ Emphasize the importance of checking in with their bodies and emotions regularly.

Emotion Quest Activity

Overview: The Emotion Quest Activity is an adventurous and educational game designed to help children recognize, understand, and express their emotions. Through a series of fun and interactive challenges, children will embark on a quest to discover different emotions and learn how to articulate and manage their feelings.

Goals

✓ Enhance emotional literacy by identifying and expressing various emotions.

✓ Develop self-awareness and empathy.

✓ Foster communication skills and emotional regulation.

✓ Encourage teamwork and cooperative learning.

Materials Needed

✓ Emotion Cards : Cards with pictures and descriptions of different emotions. Cards can be found in the resources section at the back of this book.

✓ Emotion Quest Map : A map outlining different stations or checkpoints where activities take place.

✓ Activity Supplies : Depending on the tasks, you may need markers, paper, props, or other craft supplies.

✓ Stickers or Tokens : Rewards for completing each station.

Instructions

✓ First, explain the concept of the Emotion Quest and its purpose : to explore and understand different emotions. Discuss the importance of recognizing and expressing emotions in a healthy way.

✓ Creating the Emotion Quest Map: Design a map with different stations or checkpoints, each representing a specific emotion. *The stations can consist of any emotion you have reviewed with the child, or you want them to work on. For example:

- Station 1: Happiness

- Station 2: Sadness

- Station 3: Anger

- Station 4: Fear

- Station 5: Surprise

- Station 6: Disgust

- Station 7: Love

- Station 8: Calm

Arrange the stations around the room, playground, or an outdoor area.

✓ Setting Up Stations : At each station, set up an activity that helps children explore the corresponding emotion. Examples include:

- Happiness Station : Draw or write about something that makes you happy. Share with a friend.

- Sadness Station : Think of a time when you felt sad. Draw a picture of it and discuss ways to feel better.

- Anger Station : Practice deep breathing or squeezing a stress ball to manage anger.

- Fear Station : Talk about something that scares you and how you can face it. Draw a picture of a superhero version of yourself.

- Surprise Station : Play a game that involves unexpected outcomes, like a mystery box with different items inside.

- Disgust Station : Describe or draw something you find yucky and discuss why you feel this way.

- Love Station : Create a card or write a note to someone you care about.

- Calm Station : Practice a calming activity like coloring a mandala or doing a simple yoga pose.

- ✓ Explaining the Quest : Give each child or group a copy of the Emotion Quest Map. Explain that they will visit each station, complete the activity, and collect a sticker or token for each completed task.

- ✓ Emotion Quest Map : A map outlining different stations or checkpoints where activities take place.

- ✓ Starting the Quest : Allow the children to start the quest, moving from one station to another at their own pace. Encourage them to think about and discuss their emotions as they complete each activity.

Discussion

- ✓ After completing the quest, gather the children for a group discussion.

- ✓ Ask them to share their favorite station and what they learned about their emotions.

- ✓ Discuss how understanding emotions can help them in everyday situations.

Benefits

- ✓ Emotional Literacy : Helps children recognize and name their emotions.

- ✓ Self-Awareness : Encourages reflection on personal feelings and experiences.

- ✓ Empathy : Promotes understanding and empathy by discussing different emotions.

- ✓ Communication Skills : Enhances verbal and non-verbal expression of emotions.

- ✓ Emotional Regulation : Provides strategies for managing emotions in healthy ways.

Emotion Charades

Objective: To improve recognition and understanding of emotions through expressive behaviors, enhancing emotional intelligence and communication skills in a fun and interactive way.

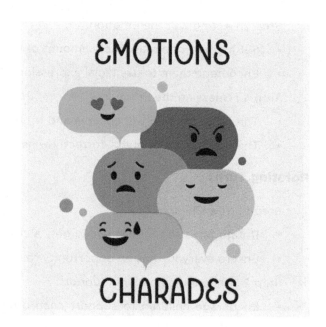

Materials Needed

- ✓ Emotion cards with illustrations (showing different emotions such as happiness, sadness, anger, surprise, fear, etc.)

- ✓ A small box or bag to hold the emotion cards

- ✓ Small rewards (e.g., stickers, small toys, certificates)

- ✓ Timer or clock

- ✓ Comfortable space for acting and observing

Emotion cards can be found at the back of this book in the resource section

Activity Steps

✓ Introduction : Explain the concept of charades and how they will be used to act out different emotions. Discuss the importance of recognizing and understanding emotions in ourselves and others.

Preparation

✓ Copy, cut, and paste the emotions cards in the resource section at the back of this book.
✓ Place the emotion cards in a box or bag.
✓ Arrange the space to allow enough room for children to act out the emotions comfortably.

Game Instructions

✓ Explain the rules of the game :

- One child will draw an emotion card from the box or bag.
- Without using words, they will act out the emotion depicted on the card.
- The other children will try to guess the emotion being portrayed.
- The first person to guess correctly will receive a small reward.

Starting the Game

✓ Step 1 : Drawing a Card.

- Select the first child to draw an emotion card from the box or bag.
- Ensure they understand the emotion they need to act out.

✓ Step 2 : Acting Out the Emotion.

- Set a timer for a reasonable amount of time (e.g., 1 minute) for the child to act out the emotion.
- Encourage them to use facial expressions, body language, and gestures to convey the emotion.

✓ Step 3 : Guessing the Emotion.

- The other children will observe and try to guess the emotion being portrayed.
- The first person to guess correctly wins.

Rotating Turns

✓ Step 1 : New Children.

- Rotate turns so that each child gets a chance to act out an emotion and guess.
- Ensure everyone has an opportunity to participate and express different emotions.

✓ Step 2 : Encouragement and Support.

- Encourage children to support each other and provide positive feedback for efforts and correct guesses.

Using Emotion Cards

✓ Step 1 : Guided Acting.

- Use emotion cards with illustrations to guide the acting and guessing process.
- Show the emotion card to the child acting out the emotion before they start.

✓ Step 2 : Visual Learning.

- After the correct guess, briefly discuss the illustration on the card and how it relates to the acted emotion.

Reflection and Discussion

✓ Step 1 : Group Reflection.

- After several rounds, gather the children for a group reflection.
- Discuss which emotions were easy or difficult to guess and why.

✓ Step 2 : Personal Experiences.

- Encourage children to share personal experiences where they felt a particular emotion and how they expressed it.

Conclusion

✓ Step 1 : Summarize the Activity.

- Summarize the importance of recognizing and understanding emotions through expressive behaviors.
- Highlight the key emotions that were acted out and discussed.

Thrilling Twist: Advanced Challenges

✓ Step 1 : Complex Emotions.

- Introduce cards with more complex or mixed emotions (e.g., confusion, excitement, disappointment).
- Challenge children to convey these emotions through more nuanced expressions.

✓ Step 2 : Group Acting.

- For older children or advanced groups, try group acting where two or more children act out a scenario involving multiple emotions.
- The rest of the group guesses the emotions involved and the scenario being portrayed.

Mindfulness Integration

✓ Step 1 : Mindful Observation.

- Teach children to observe their own and others' emotions mindfully, noticing subtle changes in expressions and body language

✓ Step 2 : Emotional Awareness.

- Encourage children to practice emotional awareness in daily life, recognizing and expressing their emotions healthily.

Additional Tips

✓ Ensure that the emotion cards are age-appropriate and easy to understand.

✓ Encourage creativity and expressiveness, emphasizing that there is no wrong way to portray an emotion.

✓ Adapt the activity for different age groups by adjusting the complexity of the emotions and scenarios.

Examples of How to Act Out Emotions

☑ Happiness

- Facial Expression : Big smile, eyes wide open, cheeks raised.

- Body Language : Jumping up and down, clapping hands, dancing, or spinning around with joy.

- Gestures : Thumbs up, high-fives, waving hands in excitement.

☑ Sadness

- Facial Expression: Frowning, eyes downcast, eyebrows drawn together.

- Body Language : Slumped shoulders, slow movements, sitting or lying down with head in hands.

- Gestures : Wiping imaginary tears, hugging oneself, covering face with hands.

☑ Anger

- Facial Expression: Furrowed brows, clenched teeth, narrowed eyes.

- Body Language : Stomping feet, clenched fists, crossing arms tightly, shaking with tension.

- Gestures : Pointing finger accusingly, throwing hands up in frustration, hitting a table (lightly).

☑ Surprise

- Facial Expression: Raised eyebrows, wide eyes, open mouth.

- Body Language : Jumping back slightly, putting hands over mouth, stepping back.

- Gestures : Clapping hands to cheeks, holding head with both hands, waving hands in front of face.

☑ Fear

- Facial Expression: Wide eyes, mouth open in a small O, eyebrows raised.

- Body Language : Huddling or shrinking back, covering face or body with arms, trembling.

- Gestures : Clutching hands together, hiding behind something, peeking out cautiously.

☑ Disgust

- Facial Expression: Nose wrinkled, upper lip raised, sticking tongue out.

- Body Language : Pulling away, turning head to the side, crossing arms over stomach.

- Gestures : Waving hand in front of nose, pushing something away, rubbing hands on clothes as if to clean them.

- **Excitement**
  - Facial Expression : Wide eyes, big smile, raised eyebrows.
  - Body Language : Jumping up and down, running in place, flapping hands.
  - Gestures : Clapping, fist-pumping, spreading arms wide.

- **Confusion**
  - Facial Expression: Furrowed brow, tilted head, mouth slightly open or pursed.
  - Body Language : Scratching head, shrugging shoulders, pacing back and forth.
  - Gestures : Spreading hands apart, pointing in different directions, looking around.

- **Boredom**
  - Facial Expression: Eyelids half-closed, mouth slightly open or closed with lips together.
  - Body Language : Slouched posture, resting head on hand, tapping fingers or foot.
  - Gestures : Yawning, looking at watch or clock, rolling eyes.

- **Shyness**
  - Facial Expression: Small smile, eyes looking down or to the side, slightly blushing cheeks.
  - Body Language : Hunching shoulders, crossing arms, taking small steps back.
  - Gestures : Twiddling fingers, playing with hair, covering part of face with hands.

- **Pride**
  - Facial Expression: Slight smile, chin up, eyes looking forward confidently.
  - Body Language : Standing tall, hands-on hips, chest out.
  - Gestures : Nodding head, patting self on the back, pointing thumbs towards self.

- **Jealousy**
  - Facial Expression: Tight lips, narrowed eyes, raised eyebrows.
  - Body Language : Crossing arms, turning body slightly away, tapping foot.
  - Gestures : Pointing finger, rolling eyes, clenching fists.

Activity: Feelings Journal

Objective: To foster regular practice of emotional expression and self-reflection by providing children with a structured yet creative outlet to explore and document their feelings.

Materials Needed

✓ Blank journals or notebooks

✓ Pens, pencils, and markers

✓ Colorful stickers and decorative items (e.g., washi tape, glitter glue)

✓ Daily prompts and questions (pre-printed or written out)

✓ Journals and pens

Activity Steps

☑ Introduction

✓ Explain the concept of a feelings journal and its purpose in helping children explore and express their emotions.

✓ Discuss the benefits of regularly reflecting on and documenting their feelings.

☑ Preparation

✓ Provide each child with a blank journal or notebook.

✓ Set up a creative station with various decorating materials such as stickers, markers, and other decorative items.

☑ Decorating the Journal:

Step 1: Personalization
- Provide each child with a blank journal or notebook.
- Set up a creative station with various decorating materials such as stickers, markers, and other decorative items.

Step 2: Creative Expression
- Provide additional decorative materials like washi tape, glitter glue, and stamps.
- Encourage them to use these materials to make their journal pages more inviting and fun.

Step 1: Providing Prompts

Provide a list of daily prompts and questions to guide the children's reflections. Examples include:

- How did you feel today? Why?
- What was the best part of your day? How did it make you feel?
- Did anything make you feel sad or upset? How did you handle it?
- Write about a time when you felt proud of yourself.
- Draw a picture of what happiness looks like to you.

Step 2: Writing and Drawing

- Encourage children to either write or draw in their journals based on the daily prompts.
- Allow them to choose how they want to express their emotions, whether through words, drawings, or a combination of both.

- **Daily Emotion Prompts**

  - How did you feel when you woke up this morning? Why do you think you felt that way?
  - What is one thing that made you smile today? Describe it.
  - Did you feel frustrated today? What happened, and how did you handle it?
  - Write about a moment when you felt calm and peaceful. What were you doing?
  - What was the most surprising thing that happened today? How did it make you feel?

- **Reflective Prompts**

  - Think of a time when you felt proud of yourself. What did you do?
  - Write about a time when you helped someone. How did it make you feel?
  - Describe a situation where you felt scared or worried. How did you overcome it?
  - Write about a time when you had a lot of fun. What were you doing, and who were you with?
  - Think about a time when you felt disappointed. What happened, and what did you learn from it?

- **Creative Expression Prompts**

  - Draw a picture of what anger looks like to you.
  - Create a comic strip about a happy moment in your life.
  - Imagine you are a superhero. What powers would you have to help people with their emotions? Draw or write about it.
  - Write a short story about a character who feels lonely. How do they find happiness?
  - Make a collage of different faces showing various emotions. Label each emotion.

- **Gratitude and Positivity Prompts**

  - Write about three things you are grateful for today. Why are they important to you?
  - Describe a time when someone was kind to you. How did it make you feel?
  - What is one positive thing you learned about yourself recently?
  - Write a thank you note to someone who made you feel special.
  - What are three things you like about yourself? Explain why.

- **Coping and Resilience Prompts**

  - Think of a difficult situation you faced recently. How did you manage it, and what helped you feel better?
  - Write about a time when you felt really angry. What did you do to calm down?
  - Describe a relaxing activity that helps you feel better when you are upset.
  - Write about a time when you had to be very patient. How did you feel afterward?
  - What are some ways you can cheer yourself up when you are feeling down?

- **Future and Goals Prompts**

  - Write about an emotion you want to understand better. Why is it important to you?
  - What are some goals you have for managing your emotions better? How will you achieve them?
  - Imagine your perfect day. What emotions would you feel, and what would you be doing?
  - Describe how you would like to handle stress in the future. What strategies will you use?
  - Write about an emotional goal you have for the next month. How will you work towards it?

- **Social and Empathy Prompts**

  - Think about a time when you saw someone else feeling sad. How did you respond, and how did it make you feel?
  - Write about a friend or family member who understands your feelings well. How do they help you?
  - Describe a time when you and a friend had a disagreement. How did you resolve it?
  - What are some ways you can show empathy to others?
  - Write about a time when you felt misunderstood. What could have helped others understand your feelings better?

- **Fun and Imagination Prompts**

  - If your feelings were an animal, what kind would they be today? Draw or write about it.
  - Imagine a world where everyone is always happy. What would it look like, and how would people behave?
  - Create a poem about a feeling you had today.
  - Write a letter to your future self about how you handle emotions now and what you hope to improve.
  - Draw a map of your "feelings land" with different areas for different emotions. Label each area and describe it.

Regular Journal Time

Step 1: Setting a Routine

- Set aside a specific time each day for children to work on their feelings journal, such as after school or before bedtime.
- Encourage consistency to help them develop the habit of regular reflection.

Step 2: Guided Reflection

- Occasionally guide the children through the process, especially if they are unsure what to write or draw.
- Offer support and encouragement to make the experience positive and productive.

Sharing and Discussion

Step 1: Optional Sharing

- Create an optional sharing time where children can share their journal entries if they feel comfortable.
- Foster a supportive environment where children can express their emotions openly and without judgment.

Step 2: Group Discussion

- Facilitate group discussions about common themes in their journal entries, such as handling difficult emotions or celebrating achievements.
- Encourage empathy and understanding among the children.

✓ Thrilling Twist: Rewards and Challenges

Step 1: Decorating Rewards

- Provide colorful stickers and markers as rewards for regular journaling.
- Encourage children to use these rewards to further decorate their journals.

Step 2: Creative Challenges

✓ Introduce creative challenges such as:
- Decorate a page with stickers that represents your feelings.
- Write a short story about a time when you felt a strong emotion.
- Create a comic strip about an emotional experience.

✓ Mindfulness and Emotional Awareness

Step 1: Mindful Writing

- Teach children mindfulness techniques to help them focus on their feelings before journaling.
- Encourage them to take deep breaths and think about their emotions before writing or drawing.

Step 2: Emotional Vocabulary

- Help children expand their emotional vocabulary by introducing new words and encouraging them to use these words in their journal entries.
- Provide examples and explanations of different emotions to help them articulate their feelings better.

✓ Reflection and Progress

Step 1: Reviewing Entries

- Periodically review the journal entries with the children to reflect on their emotional growth and changes over time.
- Celebrate their progress in understanding and expressing their emotions.

Step 2: Setting Goals

- Encourage children to set goals for their emotional well-being based on their journal reflections.
- Help them identify areas they want to improve, such as managing anger or expressing gratitude.

✓ Conclusion:

✓ Summarize the importance of regular emotional expression and self-reflection.

✓ Encourage children to continue using their feelings journal as a tool for emotional growth and self-awareness.

Additional Tips

✓ Ensure that the journaling process is always positive and pressure-free.

✓ Respect each child's privacy and only encourage sharing if they are comfortable.

✓ Adapt the activity for different age groups by simplifying or complicating the prompts as needed.

Activity: Feelings Thermometer

Objective: To help children gauge the intensity of their emotions and communicate them effectively by using a visual representation of their feelings.

FEELINGS THERMOMETER

✓ A large thermometer template (printed or drawn on a poster board). A thermometer template is included in the resources section at the back of this book.

✓ Markers or crayons

✓ Colorful stickers and decorative items (e.g., washi tape, glitter glue)

✓ Movable markers (e.g., clothespins, magnetic markers, or Velcro arrows)

✓ Journals and pens (optional)

✓ List of emotions with corresponding intensity levels

Activity Steps

☑ Introduction

✓ Explain the concept of the feelings thermometer and its purpose in helping children understand and communicate the intensity of their emotions.

✓ Discuss how recognizing different levels of emotion intensity can help in managing and expressing feelings appropriately.

☑ Preparation

✓ Provide each child with a thermometer template and decorating materials.

✓ Set up a comfortable area for the activity, with tables for decorating and space for the group discussion.

Creating the Feelings Thermometer

Step 1: Decorating the Thermometer

- Allow children to decorate their thermometer template using markers, crayons, stickers, and other decorative items.
- Encourage them to use colors and images that represent different emotions (e.g., blue for calm, red for anger).

Step 2: Labeling Intensity Levels

- Help children label different sections of the thermometer with varying levels of emotional intensity (e.g., calm, upset, very angry).
- Provide examples of what each level might feel like or look like.

Using the Feelings Thermometer

Step 1: Introducing the Movable Markers

- Show children how to use the movable markers to indicate their current emotional intensity.
- Explain that they can move the marker up and down the thermometer as their emotions change throughout the day.

Step 2: Practicing with Scenarios

- Present different scenarios and ask children to move their marker to the appropriate level on the thermometer.
- Example scenarios: "You lost your favorite toy," "You got a good grade on a test," "You had an argument with a friend."

Regular Check-Ins

Step 1: Daily Use

- Encourage children to use the feelings thermometer regularly to check in with their emotions, especially during transition times (e.g., after school, before bedtime).
- Allow them to adjust their marker as needed throughout the day.

Step 2: Guided Reflections

- Periodically guide the children in reflecting on their emotional intensity. Ask questions like:
    - "What happened that made you feel this way?"
    - "What can you do to move your marker down (if feeling intense negative emotions)?"
    - "How does it feel when your marker is at the calm level?"

Thrilling Twist: Real Thermometer Template

Step 1: Using a Real Thermometer Template

- Provide a real thermometer template (either a printed image or a plastic model).
- Let children use colors and stickers to decorate it, assigning different emotions to different temperature levels.

Step 2: Interactive Decorating

- Encourage children to be creative with their decorations, using colors that represent how they feel at each level.
- Add fun elements like glitter glue, patterned washi tape, or themed stickers (e.g., sun for happy, storm cloud for angry).

Sharing and Discussion

Step 1: Group Sharing

- Create opportunities for children to share their feelings thermometer with the group.
- Encourage them to explain their choices for colors and decorations.

Step 2: Emotional Discussions

- Facilitate discussions about how different emotions feel and how they can manage emotions that are at the higher intensity levels.
- Encourage empathy and support among the children as they share their experiences.

Reflection and Journaling (Optional)

Step 1 : Journaling Prompts

- Provide journaling prompts for children to reflect on their feelings and the use of the thermometer.
- Example prompts: "How did I feel today? Where was my marker most of the time? What can I do to help myself feel calmer?"

Step 2: Tracking Progress

- Encourage children to track their emotional intensity over time, noting any patterns or changes.
- Use the journal to discuss strategies for maintaining or achieving a calmer state.

☑ Conclusion

✓ Summarize the importance of recognizing and communicating the intensity of emotions.

✓ Encourage children to continue using their feelings thermometer as a tool for emotional self-awareness and regulation.

Additional Tips

✓ Ensure that the feelings thermometer is age-appropriate and easy to understand.

✓ Reinforce the idea that all emotions are valid, and it is okay to feel different intensities.

✓ Adapt the activity for different age groups by simplifying or adding complexity to the thermometer and prompts.

Activity: Feelings Volcano

Objective: To help children understand how emotions can build up and erupt like a volcano, and to provide them with a visual and interactive tool to gauge and communicate the intensity of their feelings.

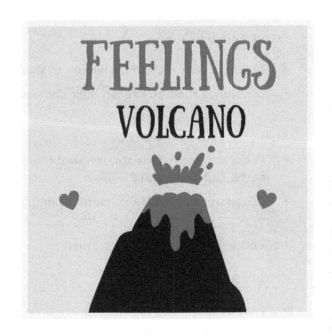

Materials Needed

✓ A large volcano template (printed or drawn on a poster board)

✓ Markers or crayons

✓ Colorful stickers and decorative items (e.g., washi tape, glitter glue)

✓ Movable markers (e.g., clothespins, magnetic markers, or Velcro arrows)

✓ Journals and pens (optional)

✓ List of emotions with corresponding intensity levels

Activity Steps

☑ Introduction

✓ Explain the concept of the feelings volcano and how it represents the way emotions can build up and erupt if not managed properly.

✓ Discuss how recognizing and expressing emotions before they reach the eruption point can help in managing feelings effectively.

✪ Preparation

✓ Provide each child with a volcano template and decorating materials.

✓ Set up a comfortable area for the activity, with tables for decorating and space for group discussion.

✪ Creating the Feelings Volcano

Step 1: Decorating the Volcano

- Allow children to decorate their volcano template using markers, crayons, stickers, and other decorative items.

- Encourage them to use colors and images that represent different emotions (e.g., blue for calm, red for anger).

Step 2: Labeling Intensity Levels

- Help children label different sections of the volcano with varying levels of emotional intensity, from the base (calm) to the top (erupting).

- Provide examples of what each level might feel like or look like, such as:

  - **Base:** Calm and relaxed

  - **Middle:** Upset or frustrated

  - **Top:** Very angry or about to erupt

✪ Using the Feelings Volcano

Step 1: Introducing the Movable Markers

- Show children how to use the movable markers to indicate their current emotional intensity.

- Explain that they can move the marker up and down the volcano as their emotions change throughout the day.

- Use any item as a 'marker.' The purpose is to move that item up or down depending on feelings.

Step 2: Practicing with Scenarios

- Present different scenarios and ask children to move their marker to the appropriate level on the volcano.

- Example scenarios: "You lost your favorite toy," "You got a good grade on a test," "You had an argument with a friend."

☑ Regular Check-Ins

Step 1: Daily Use

- Encourage children to use the feelings volcano regularly to check in with their emotions, especially during transition times (e.g., after school, before bedtime).

- Allow them to adjust their marker as needed throughout the day.

Step 2: Guided Reflections

- Periodically guide the children in reflecting on their emotional intensity. Ask questions like:

    - "What happened that made you feel this way?"

    - "What can you do to move your marker down (if feeling intense negative emotions)?"

    - "How does it feel when your marker is at the base level?"

☑ Thrilling Twist: Real Volcano Template

Step 1: Using a Real Volcano Template

- Provide a real volcano template (either a printed image or a 3D model).

- Let children use colors and stickers to decorate it, assigning different emotions to different levels.

Step 2: Interactive Decorating

- Encourage children to be creative with their decorations, using colors that represent how they feel at each level.

- Add fun elements like glitter glue, patterned washi tape, or themed stickers (e.g., flames for anger, calm waves for relaxed).

Activity: Feelings Fortune Teller

Materials Needed

✓ Square sheets of paper (one per child)

✓ Markers or crayons

✓ Stickers and decorative items (optional)

✓ List of emotions and feelings

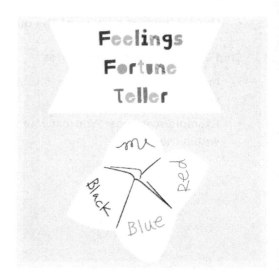

Steps to Fold the Fortune Teller

✓ Prepare the Square Paper

✓ Ensure each child has a square sheet of paper. If starting with a rectangular sheet, you can make it square by folding one corner diagonally across to the opposite edge and cutting off the excess strip.

✓ Fold Diagonally

Step 1: First Diagonal Fold

- Fold the square paper in half diagonally to form a triangle. Crease well, then unfold.

Step 2: Second Diagonal Fold

- Fold the paper in half diagonally the other way to form another triangle. Crease well, then unfold. You should now have an X crease on your paper.

✓ Fold Corners to the Center

Step 1: First Corner Fold

- Take one corner of the square and fold it into the center where the diagonal creases intersect. Crease well.

Step 2: Continue Folding Corners

- Repeat this process for the remaining three corners, folding each into the center to create a smaller square.

✓ Flip and Repeat

Step 1: Flip the Paper Over

- Flip the paper over so that the folded flaps are facing down.

Step 2: Fold Corners to Center Again

- Fold each corner into the center again, creating an even smaller square.

✓ Fold into Shape

Step 1: Fold in Half

- Fold the paper in half horizontally to make a rectangle, then crease and unfold.

Step 2: Fold Corners to Center Again

- Fold each corner into the center again, creating an even smaller square.

☑ Form the Fortune Teller

Step 1: Create the Pockets

- With the square facing up, gently lift the four flaps in the center to form pockets where fingers can fit.

Step 2: Insert Fingers

- Insert your index fingers and thumbs into the four pockets. Push your fingers together, and the fortune teller will start to take shape.

Decorating and Labeling

☑ Outside Flaps

✓ **Numbers:** On the outside flaps, write the numbers 1 through 8 (one number on each triangle). These numbers will be used to open and close the fortune teller during the game.

☑ Inside Flaps

✓ **Colors or Symbols:** Open the fortune teller to reveal the inner flaps. Write different colors or symbols on these flaps. Each color or symbol will correspond to a set of emotions written inside.

☑ Inner Sections

✓ **Emotions:** Open the flaps to reveal the inner sections where the fortunes are usually written. In each section, write different emotions and feelings. For example:

- Happy
- Sad
- Angry
- Excited
- Nervous
- Proud
- Confused
- Surprised

Example of Labeling

☑ Outside Flaps

✓ Number the outside flaps from 1 to 8

☑ Inside Flaps

✓ On the inside flaps, write colors like red, blue, green, yellow, or symbols like stars, hearts, smiley faces, and lightning bolts.

- ☑ Inner Sections

 - ✓ Write one emotion in each inner section, ensuring a variety of feelings are represented.

Using the Fortune Teller

- ☑ Choosing Numbers

 - ✓ One child asks their partner to choose a number. They open and close the fortune teller that many times.

- ☑ Choosing Colors/Symbols

 - ✓ The partner then chooses a color or symbol. The first child spells out the color or opens and closes the fortune teller according to the symbol.

- ☑ Revealing Emotions

 - ✓ The partner chooses another number, and the first child opens the flap to reveal the emotion written inside.
 - ✓ Discuss the emotion revealed, asking questions about personal experiences, physical sensations, and strategies for managing that emotion.

Additional Tips

- ✓ Practice folding the fortune teller a few times to ensure you can guide the children effectively.
- ✓ Make sure the children understand each step before moving on to the next.
- ✓ Encourage creativity in decorating the fortune teller to make it a fun and personalized activity.

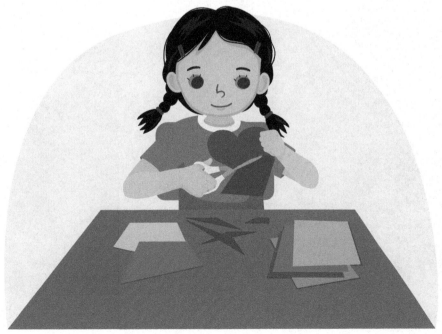

CHAPTER - 4

FeeL The WORLD

Skin Sensations

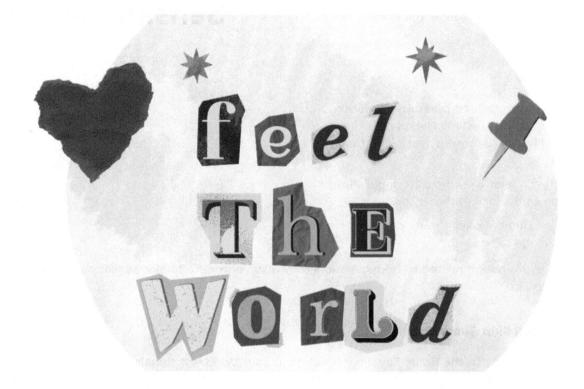

Welcome to the fascinating world of skin sensations! Your skin is your body's largest organ and a powerful sensory system that helps you interact with the world around you. In this chapter, we will explore how your skin senses touch, temperature, pressure, pain, and more. You will learn how to decode these sensations and understand what they mean.

Understanding Skin Sensations

Skin Anatomy and Sensory Receptors

To help children understand how emotions can build up and erupt like a volcano, and to provide them with a visual and interactive tool to gauge and communicate the intensity of their feelings.

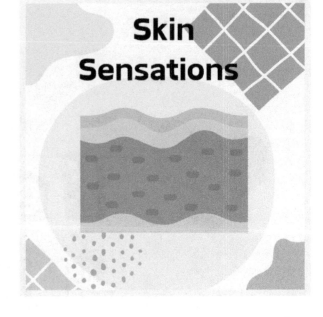

Sensory Receptors

✓ Mechanoreceptors: Detect pressure, vibration, and texture. Examples include Merkel cells (light touch) and Meissner's corpuscles (light touch and texture).

✓ Thermoreceptors: Sense changes in temperature. They include cold and warm receptors.

✓ Nociceptors: Detect pain from damage or potential damage to tissues.

✓ Proprioceptors: Although related to body position, they also contribute to skin sensations, especially in joints and muscles.

The Science Behind Skin Sensations

✓ How Sensations Travel to the Brain: Sensory receptors in your skin send signals through the peripheral nerves to the spinal cord and then to the brain. The brain processes these signals in the somatosensory cortex, allowing you to perceive different sensations.

Types of Sensory Receptors

✓ There are several types of sensory receptors, each specialized for detecting different types of stimuli. These receptors can be broadly categorized into the following types:

✓ Mechanoreceptors: Detect mechanical changes such as pressure, vibration, and stretch. Found in the skin, muscles, tendons, and internal organs.

- **Pacinian Corpuscles:** Respond to deep pressure and vibration

- **Meissner's Corpuscles:** Sensitive to light touch and changes in texture.

- **Merkel Cells:** Detect sustained pressure and texture.

- **Ruffini Endings:** Respond to skin stretch and contribute to the sense of finger position and movement.

- ☑ Thermoreceptors: Detect changes in temperature. Primarily located in the skin, as well as in the hypothalamus (which monitors body's internal temperature).

  - Cold Receptors: Activated by cool temperatures.

  - Warm Receptors: Activated by warm temperatures.

  - Thermoreceptive Nerve Endings: Detect a range of temperature changes.

- ☑ Nociceptors: Detect painful stimuli or potentially damaging stimuli. Found in the skin, muscles, joints, and internal organs.

  - Mechanical Nociceptors: Respond to physical damage like cutting or crushing.

  - Thermal Nociceptors: Activated by extreme temperatures.

  - Chemical Nociceptors: Respond to chemical stimuli such as those from inflammation.

- ☑ Chemoreceptors: Detect chemical stimuli. Found in the nose, tongue, blood vessels, and brain.

  - Olfactory Receptors: Detect smells.

  - Gustatory Receptors: Detect tastes.

- ☑ Photoreceptors: Detect light. Found in the retina of the eye

  - Rods: Sensitive to low light levels and important for night vision.

  - Cones: Detect color and are important for day vision and color discrimination.

*This is a sample list. There are many more receptors in your body!

How Sensory Receptors Work

✓ When a sensory receptor is stimulated by an appropriate stimulus, it undergoes a change in its membrane potential. This change, called a receptor potential, can generate an action potential if it is strong enough. The action potential travels along sensory neurons to the central nervous system (CNS), where it is processed and interpreted. The brain then translates these electrical signals into recognizable sensations.

The Role of the Nervous System

✓ The peripheral nervous system (PNS) includes all the nerves outside the brain and spinal cord. The PNS communicates sensory information to the central nervous system (CNS), which consists of the brain and spinal cord. Each sensation travels via a specific pathway to reach the brain. The sense of smell travels DIRECTLY to the brain first and then it is sent to other brain regions. That's why smell is so powerful!

Importance in Interoception

✓ Interoception relies heavily on sensory receptors to monitor the internal state of your body. For example, mechanoreceptors in the stomach walls can detect when the stomach is full, while chemoreceptors in the blood can detect changes in oxygen and carbon dioxide levels, signaling the need to breathe. This all occurs automatically. Understanding and responding to internal signals helps maintain your body's balance (homeostasis) and overall well-being.

Find A Texture

Description

Go on a hunt around your house or classroom to find objects with different textures (smooth, rough, soft, hard). Close your eyes and feel each object, then describe the texture and guess what the object is.

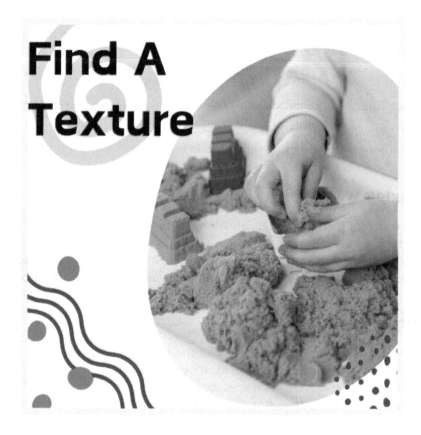

TEXTURE TYPE	DESCRIPTION	WHAT I FOUND
Smooth	Sleek, even, polished	
Rough	Coarse, bumpy, gritty	
Soft	Fluffy, plush, velvety	
Hard	Rigid, solid, firm	
Sticky	Adhesive, tacky, gluey	
Slippery	Slick, greasy, oily	
Fuzzy	Woolly, hairy, downy	
Grainy	Sandy, granular, gritty	
Crumbly	Fragile, breakable, brittle	
Spongy	Squishy, porous, absorbent	
Prickly	Spiky, thorny, barbed	
Slimy	Mucous, slippery, slick	
Metallic	Shiny, cold, steely	
Rubbery	Elastic, flexible, springy	

Use the chart above or make your own

Goal : Develop awareness of different textures and how your skin perceives them.

Temperature Detective

To develop children's ability to detect and describe temperature variations on their skin, enhancing their interoceptive awareness and understanding of how temperature sensations are perceived by the body.

Materials Needed

✓ Ice cubes

✓ Warm water

✓ Room temperature water

✓ Small bowls or cups

✓ Towels

✓ Timer or clock

✓ Notepad and pen for each child

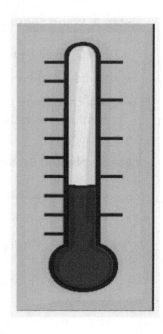

Activity Steps

✅ Introduction

✓ Explain the importance of interoception and how temperature detection is a key aspect of interoceptive awareness.

✓ Discuss how our skin can detect a wide range of temperatures and the body's responses to these sensations.

✅ Preparation

✓ Set up three small bowls or cups filled with warm water, ice-cold water, and room temperature water.

✓ Ensure that the warm water is comfortably warm, not hot, to prevent any risk of burns or discomfort.

✅ Initial Observation

✓ Have children sit comfortably and place their hands on their laps.

✓ Ask them to close their eyes and take a few deep breaths to relax and center their attention on their hands.

✅ Temperature Exploration

Step 1: Cold Sensation

- Ask children to dip one hand into the bowl of ice-cold water for 10-15 seconds.

- Remove the hand and place it on a towel to dry.

- Encourage children to focus on the sensations in their hand and describe them (e.g., tingling, numbness, cold).

Step 2: Warm Sensation

- Next, have children dip the same hand into the bowl of warm water for 10-15 seconds.

- Remove the hand and place it on a towel to dry.

- Ask children to notice the change in sensation and describe how their hand feels now (e.g., warmth, comfort, relaxation).

Step 3: Neutral Sensation

- Finally, have children dip their hand into the bowl of room temperature water for 10-15 seconds.

- Remove the hand and place it on a towel to dry.

- Encourage them to describe the sensations and compare them with previous experiences.

✅ Comparative Exploration

✓ Repeat the process with the other hand, but in a different order (e.g., start with warm water, then ice-cold, and finish with room temperature).

✓ This helps children detect subtle differences and understand how initial temperature exposure affects subsequent sensations.

✅ Sensory Journaling

✓ Provide time for children to journal their experiences and observations.

✓ Ask them to note any differences in sensations between the two hands, how quickly their skin adapted to temperature changes, and any unexpected feelings.

✅ Group Discussion

✓ Facilitate a group discussion where children can share their findings and reflect on their experiences.

✓ Encourage them to discuss how their perception of temperature may vary in different environments or situations.

✅ Mindfulness Integration

✓ Guide children through a brief mindfulness exercise focused on temperature sensations.

✓ Have them close their eyes and imagine placing their hands in different temperature environments, paying close attention to the sensations that arise.

✅ Conclusion

✓ Summarize the importance of being aware of temperature sensations and how this practice can enhance interoceptive awareness.

✓ Encourage children to practice temperature detection exercises in their daily lives to build a stronger connection with their bodily sensations.

Additional Tips

✓ Ensure all temperatures used are safe and comfortable for children.

✓ Encourage children to take their time and fully engage with each sensation.

✓ Adapt the activity for different age groups or sensitivity levels by adjusting the duration of exposure and temperature intensity.

Feather and Stone Challenge

Objective: To enhance children's sensitivity to different types of pressure and texture, fostering a deeper understanding of interoceptive awareness through the contrasting sensations of light and heavy objects.

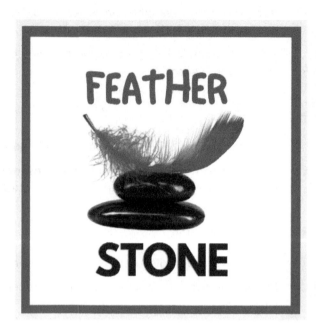

Materials Needed

✓ Feathers

✓ Smooth stones or pebbles (small enough to be held comfortably in one hand)

✓ Blindfolds (optional)

✓ Soft pillows or mats for comfort

✓ Journals and pens

Activity Steps

✓ Introduction

✓ Explain the concept of interoception and the importance of being aware of different sensations on the skin.

✓ Discuss how the skin can detect various pressures and textures, contributing to our overall body awareness.

✓ Preparation

✓ Provide each child with a feather and a smooth stone.

✓ Ensure the stones are clean and smooth to prevent any discomfort or injury.

✓ Initial Sensory Awareness

✓ Ask children to sit or lie down in a comfortable position on mats or pillows.

✓ Encourage them to close their eyes or use blindfolds to enhance their focus on the sensations.

✓ Light Touch Exploration

Step 1: Feather Sensation

- Guide children to gently brush the feather against their skin, starting with their hands and moving to other parts of their body, such as their arms, face, and neck.

- Ask them to pay close attention to the light, tickling sensation and note any differences in sensitivity across various body parts.

Step 2: Feather Mindfulness

- Encourage children to slow down and take deep breaths, focusing on the feather's delicate touch.
- Ask them to describe the sensations in their journal, noting any areas that felt particularly sensitive or relaxing.

Heavy Pressure Exploration

Step 1: Stone Sensation

- Guide children to hold the smooth stone in one hand, feeling its weight and texture.
- Ask them to gently press the stone against different parts of their body, starting with their palms and moving to their arms, legs, and shoulders.
- Encourage them to notice the contrast between the light feather touch and the heavier stone pressure.

Step 2: Stone Mindfulness

- Have children take a few moments to focus on the sensations created by the stone, taking note of how their skin and muscles respond to the pressure.
- Ask them to describe these sensations in their journal, comparing them with the feather's touch.

Combining Sensations

Step 1: Alternating Sensations

- Guide children to alternate between the feather and the stone, first brushing the feather against their skin and then pressing the stone.
- Encourage them to notice how quickly their skin adapts to the changing sensations and any new observations that arise.

Step 2: Full Body Exploration

- Ask children to explore different parts of their body with both the feather and the stone, paying attention to areas that might feel different than others (e.g., the back of the neck versus the forearm).

Sensory Journaling

- Provide time for children to journal their experiences and reflections.
- Ask them to note any new insights about their body's sensitivity, how different parts of their body responded to the feather and stone, and any emotional responses they experienced.

- ☑ Group Discussion

  ✓ Facilitate a group discussion where children can share their findings and reflect on their experiences.

  ✓ Encourage them to discuss how the contrasting sensations of light and heavy objects can enhance their interoceptive awareness.

- ☑ Mindfulness Integration

  ✓ Guide children through a brief mindfulness exercise focused on recalling the sensations of the feather and stone.

  ✓ Have them visualize the feather's light touch and the stone's heavy pressure, noticing any lingering sensations or memories.

- ☑ Conclusion

  ✓ Summarize the importance of being aware of different types of pressure and texture sensations.

  ✓ Encourage children to incorporate similar sensory exploration activities into their daily lives to build a stronger connection with their bodily sensations.

Additional Tips

✓ Ensure that children are comfortable, and that the environment is quiet and free from distractions.

✓ Encourage children to take their time and fully engage with each sensation, emphasizing that there is no right or wrong way to experience the activities.

✓ Adapt the activity for different age groups or sensitivity levels by adjusting the intensity and duration of the sensory exploration.

Activity: Pinch and Rubber Band Snap for Pain Awareness

Objective : To help children develop a deeper understanding of pain sensations through controlled, mild pain stimuli, and to enhance their ability to recognize and describe these sensations as part of their interoceptive awareness practice.

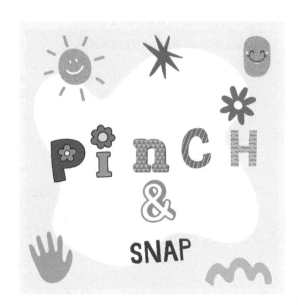

Materials Needed

✓ Rubber bands (sized to fit comfortably around a wrist or finger without cutting off circulation)

✓ Journals and pens

✓ Comfortable seating or mats

✓ Soft pillows or cushions for support

Activity Steps

✔ Introduction

✔ Explain the concept of interoception and its importance in recognizing and understanding pain sensations.

✔ Discuss how controlled, mild pain stimuli can help improve awareness of how the body experiences and responds to pain.

✔ Preparation

✔ Create a comfortable and calm environment for the activity.

✔ Provide each child with a rubber band and a journal.

✔ Initial Relaxation

✔ Ask children to sit comfortably and take a few deep breaths to relax and center their attention on their bodies.

✔ Guide them through a brief relaxation exercise to release any initial tension.

✔ Pinch Exploration

Step 1: Gentle Pinch

- Instruct children to gently pinch the skin on the back of their hand, arm, or leg.
- Ask them to hold the pinch for a few seconds and then release.
- Encourage them to focus on the sensation of the pinch, noting the intensity, location, and type of pain (e.g., sharp, dull, throbbing).

Step 2: Repeat and Observe

- Have children repeat the gentle pinch on different areas of their body, such as the forearm, upper arm, and thigh.
- Ask them to observe any differences in pain sensation between these areas.

Step 3: Journaling

- Provide time for children to journal their observations, describing the sensations they experienced during the pinching activity.

☑ Rubber Band Snap Exploration

Step 1: Rubber Band Placement

- Instruct children to place a rubber band around their wrist or finger, ensuring it is not too tight.
- Ask them to gently pull the rubber band away from their skin and then release it to create a mild snapping sensation.

Step 2: Focus on Sensation

- Encourage children to focus on the sensation of the rubber band snap, noting the intensity, location, and type of pain.
- Have them repeat the snapping action a few times, paying close attention to any changes in sensation.

Step 3: Journaling

- Provide time for children to journal their observations, describing the sensations they experienced during the rubber band snap activity.

☑ Mindfulness and Pain Management

Step 1: Deep Breathing

- Guide children through a deep breathing exercise, encouraging them to focus on their breath and any lingering sensations of pain.
- Teach them to use deep breathing to manage and alleviate pain sensations.

Step 2: Visualization

- Lead children in a visualization exercise, asking them to imagine the pain as a specific shape or color.
- Encourage them to visualize the pain changing or dissolving with each breath.

☑ Mindfulness and Pain Management

✓ Facilitate a group discussion where children can share their experiences and insights.

✓ Encourage them to discuss how the pinch and rubber band snap activities affected their pain awareness and any new understanding they gained about their body's response to pain.

☑ Conclusion

✓ Summarize the importance of being aware of pain sensations and how these controlled activities can help improve interoceptive awareness.

✓ Encourage children to use these techniques mindfully and to practice pain awareness exercises in a safe and controlled manner.

Additional Tips

✓ Emphasize the importance of keeping the pain stimuli mild and controlled to prevent any harm or discomfort.

✓ Ensure children understand that the goal is to explore pain awareness, not to cause significant pain or distress.

✓ Adapt the activity for different sensitivity levels, providing alternative methods if needed (e.g., using a softer rubber band or a gentler pinch).

Mystery Touch Box

Activity: Mystery Touch Box

Objective: To enhance tactile exploration skills and improve the ability to identify objects through touch alone, fostering a deeper understanding of texture, size, and shape as part of interoceptive awareness.

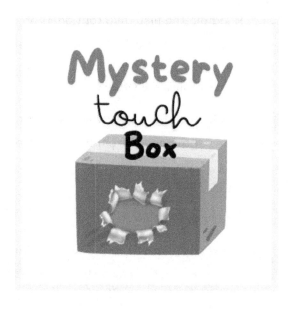

Materials Needed

✓ A large cardboard box with a hole cut in one side (big enough for a hand to fit through comfortably)

✓ A variety of objects with different textures, sizes, and shapes (e.g., a sponge, a small toy, a piece of fabric, a coin, a smooth stone, a pinecone, a rubber ball, a key)

✓ A blindfold (optional)

✓ Journals and pens

Activity Steps

☑ Introduction

✓ Explain the concept of tactile exploration and its importance in interoceptive awareness.

✓ Discuss how identifying objects through touch alone can enhance sensory perception and body awareness.

☑ Preparation

✓ Create a comfortable environment for the activity.

✓ Place the box with the hole on a table or on the floor where children can easily reach it.

✓ Ensure the box is opaque and that children cannot see inside.

Initial Relaxation

✓ Ask children to sit comfortably around the box.

✓ Guide them through a brief relaxation exercise to help them focus on their tactile sensations.

Mystery Touch Box Exploration

Step 1: Introducing the Box

- Explain how the Mystery Touch Box works and the purpose of the activity.
- Demonstrate reaching into the box and feeling an object without looking.

Step 2: First Exploration

- Blindfold the first child (optional) or simply ask them to close their eyes.
- Have the child reach into the box, feel an object, and describe its texture, size, and shape aloud.

Step 3: Guessing the Object

- Ask the child to guess what the object is based on their tactile observations.
- Remove the object from the box to reveal it and discuss the accuracy of their guess

Rotating Turns

Step 1: Multiple Children

- Allow each child to take a turn reaching into the box and feeling an object.
- Ensure each child has a chance to describe and guess at least one object.

Step 2: Varying Objects

- Change the objects in the box for each child to ensure a variety of textures, sizes, and shapes.
- Encourage children to pay close attention to the details they feel.

Comparative Exploration

Step 1: Discussing Differences

- After all children have taken their turns, facilitate a discussion about the different objects and how they were perceived.
- Encourage children to compare their tactile experiences and discuss any challenges they faced in identifying the objects.

Step 2: Observing Reactions

- Ask children to reflect on how their skin and tactile senses responded to different textures, sizes, and shapes.
- Encourage them to note any patterns or preferences in their tactile perceptions.

Sensory Journaling

✓ Provide time for children to journal their observations and reflections.

✓ Ask them to describe the sensations they experienced, the objects they identified, and any new insights they gained about their tactile perception.

Mindfulness and Tactile Awareness

Step 1: Guided Visualization

- Lead children through a guided visualization exercise, asking them to imagine the textures, sizes, and shapes of the objects they felt.
- Encourage them to focus on the tactile sensations and how their body responds in their mind's eye.

Step 2: Sensory Integration

- Teach children techniques for integrating tactile awareness into their daily lives, such as mindful touching of everyday objects or focusing on textures during daily activities.

Group Discussion

✓ Facilitate a group discussion where children can share their experiences and insights.

✓ Encourage them to discuss how the Mystery Touch Box activity enhanced their tactile exploration skills and any new understanding they gained about their body's response to touch.

Conclusion

✓ Summarize the importance of tactile exploration and how identifying objects through touch can enhance interoceptive awareness.

✓ Encourage children to practice tactile awareness exercises regularly to build a stronger connection with their bodily sensations.

Additional Tips

✓ Ensure the objects in the box are safe to touch and free from sharp edges or points.

✓ Encourage children to take their time and fully explore each object before making a guess.

✓ Adapt the activity for different age groups or sensitivity levels by selecting appropriate objects and adjusting the level of difficulty.

Activity: Ice and Heat Sensation Exploration

Objective: To help children understand how thermoreceptors react to different temperatures and enhance their interoceptive awareness by observing and comparing the body's response to cold and warm sensations.

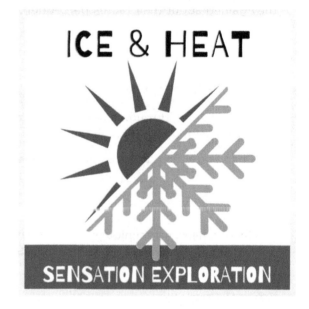

Materials Needed

✓ Ice cubes

✓ Cool packs

✓ Warm washcloths (ensure they are warm but not hot to prevent burns)

✓ Warm packs

✓ Essential oils (optional)

✓ Towels

✓ Timer or clock

✓ Journals and pens

Activity Steps

◉ Introduction

✓ Explain the role of thermoreceptors in the skin and how they help us detect temperature changes.

✓ Discuss the importance of understanding the body's response to different temperatures as part of interoceptive awareness.

◉ Preparation

✓ Create a comfortable environment for the activity.

✓ Provide each child with an ice cube, a warm washcloth, and a journal for recording observations.

☑ Initial Relaxation

✓ Ask children to sit or lie down comfortably.

✓ Guide them through a brief relaxation exercise to help them focus on their body's sensations.

☑ Ice Sensation Exploration

Step 1: Applying the Ice Cube or Cool Pack

- Instruct children to take an ice cube and place it on a specific part of their body, such as the back of their hand, forearm, or inner wrist.
- Ask them to hold the ice cube in place and observe how long it takes to feel the cold sensation.

Step 2: Focusing on Sensation

- Encourage children to focus on the intensity and spread of the cold sensation.
- Ask them to note any changes in sensation over time, such as numbness or tingling.

Step 3: Journaling

- Provide time for children to journal their observations, describing the sensations they experienced, how quickly they felt the cold, and any differences between body parts.

☑ Heat Sensation Exploration

Step 1: Applying the Warm Washcloth or Warm Pack

- Instruct children to take a warm washcloth and place it on a different part of their body, such as the opposite hand, forearm, or inner wrist.
- Ask them to hold the washcloth in place and observe how long it takes to feel the warmth.

Step 2: Focusing on Sensation

- Encourage children to focus on the intensity and spread of the warm sensation.
- Ask them to note any changes in sensation over time, such as relaxation or increased warmth.

Step 3: Journaling

- Provide time for children to journal their observations, describing the sensations they experienced, how quickly they felt the warmth, and any differences between body parts.

☑ Comparative Exploration

Step 1: Alternating Sensations

- Ask children to alternate between the ice cube and the warm washcloth, placing them on the same body part (e.g., switching between the back of the hand and the forearm).
- Encourage them to compare the sensations of cold and warmth, noting the body's reactions and any differences in sensitivity.

Step 2: Observing Reactions

- Have children observe how their skin and body react to alternating temperatures, such as changes in skin color, goosebumps, or muscle tension.

Step 3: Journaling

- Provide time for children to journal their comparative observations, describing the differences in sensations, the body's responses, and any new insights they gained.

☑ Mindfulness and Temperature Awareness

Step 1: Guided Visualization

- Lead children through a guided visualization exercise, asking them to imagine the sensations of ice and warmth on different parts of their body.
- Encourage them to focus on the sensations and how their body responds in their mind's eye.

Step 2: Breathing Techniques

- Teach children deep breathing techniques to help manage and alleviate any discomfort from the temperature changes.
- Encourage them to practice the techniques while focusing on the sensations of cold and warmth.

Step 3: Essential Oils (Optional)

- If using essential oils, guide children to apply a small amount of diluted essential oil to the uncomfortable area and gently massage it in.
- Encourage them to focus on the combined sensations of the massage and the scent of the oil.

✅ Group Discussion

✓ Facilitate a group discussion where children can share their experiences and insights.

✓ Encourage them to discuss how the different temperatures affected their body awareness and any new understanding they gained about their body's response to temperature changes.

✅ Conclusion

✓ Summarize the importance of being aware of temperature sensations and how understanding thermoreceptors can enhance interoceptive awareness.

✓ Encourage children to incorporate temperature awareness exercises into their daily lives to build a stronger connection with their bodily sensations.

Additional Tips

✓ Ensure that the warm washcloths are not too hot to avoid burns.

✓ Emphasize the importance of observing the sensations mindfully and not rushing the process.

✓ Adapt the activity for different sensitivity levels, providing alternative methods if needed (e.g., using slightly cooler or warmer temperatures).

✓ Ensure that children are comfortable, and that the environment is quiet and free from distractions.

✓ Emphasize the importance of listening to their bodies and not pushing themselves beyond their comfort limits.

✓ Adapt the activity for different pain levels and sensitivities, providing alternative techniques as needed.

Pressure Pathways

Activity: Pressure Pathways

Objective: To help children understand how mechanoreceptors respond to varying levels of pressure and to observe how different parts of the body perceive pressure differently, enhancing interoceptive awareness.

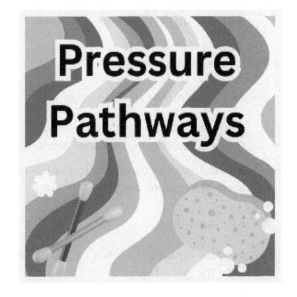

Materials Needed

✓ Soft balls (e.g., foam balls or stress balls)

✓ Pencil erasers

✓ Sponges

✓ Cotton swabs

✓ Journals and pens

✓ Comfortable seating or mats

✓ Soft pillows or cushions for support

Activity Steps

○ Introduction

✓ Explain the role of mechanoreceptors in the skin and how they help us detect pressure.

✓ Discuss the importance of understanding how different levels of pressure are perceived by various parts of the body as part of interoceptive awareness.

○ Preparation

✓ Create a comfortable environment for the activity.

✓ Provide each child with a soft ball, a pencil with an eraser, a cotton swab, and a journal.

○ Initial Relaxation

✓ Ask children to sit or lie down comfortably.

✓ Guide them through a brief relaxation exercise to help them focus on their body's sensations.

○ Soft Ball Exploration

Step 1: Applying the Soft Ball

- Instruct children to gently press the soft ball against different parts of their body, such as the palm, forearm, thigh, and back of the neck.

- Ask them to focus on the sensation of the soft ball pressing against their skin and describe the level of pressure they feel.

Step 2: Journaling

- Provide time for children to journal their observations, describing the sensations they experienced with the soft ball, noting any differences between body parts.

○ Pencil Eraser Exploration

Step 1: Applying the Pencil Eraser

- Instruct children to gently press the pencil eraser against different parts of their body, such as the fingertips, forearm, shoulder, and ankle.

- Ask them to focus on the sensation of the pencil eraser pressing against their skin and describe the level of pressure they feel.

Step 2: Journaling

- Provide time for children to journal their observations, describing the sensations they experienced with the pencil eraser, noting any differences between body parts.

Cotton Swab Exploration

Step 1: Applying the Cotton Swab

- Instruct children to gently press the cotton swab against different parts of their body, such as the wrist, back of the hand, cheek, and collarbone.
- Ask them to focus on the sensation of the cotton swab pressing against their skin and describe the level of pressure they feel.

Step 2: Journaling

- Provide time for children to journal their observations, describing the sensations they experienced with the cotton swab, noting any differences between body parts.

Comparative Exploration

Step 1: Alternating Objects

- Ask children to alternate between the soft ball, pencil eraser, and cotton swab on the same body part (e.g., switching between the palm and the forearm).
- Encourage them to compare the sensations of the different objects, noting the body's reactions and any differences in sensitivity.

Step 2: Observing Reactions

- Have children observe how their skin and body react to the varying levels of pressure, such as changes in skin color, tension, or relaxation.

Step 3: Journaling

- Provide time for children to journal their comparative observations, describing the differences in sensations, the body's responses, and any new insights they gained.

Mindfulness and Pressure Awareness

Step 1: Guided Visualization

- Lead children through a guided visualization exercise, asking them to imagine the sensations of the soft ball, pencil eraser, and cotton swab on different parts of their body.
- Encourage them to focus on the sensations and how their body responds in their mind's eye.

Step 2: Breathing Techniques

- Teach children deep breathing techniques to help manage and alleviate any discomfort from the pressure changes.
- Encourage them to practice these techniques while focusing on the sensations of different pressures.

- ☑ Group Discussion

- ✓ Facilitate a group discussion where children can share their experiences and insights.

- ✓ Encourage them to discuss how the different levels of pressure affected their body awareness and any new understanding they gained about their body's response to pressure changes.

- ☑ Conclusion

- ✓ Summarize the importance of being aware of pressure sensations and how understanding mechanoreceptors can enhance interoceptive awareness.
- ✓ Encourage children to incorporate pressure awareness exercises into their daily lives to build a stronger connection with their bodily sensations.

Additional Tips

- ✓ Ensure that children are comfortable, and that the environment is quiet and free from distractions.

- ✓ Emphasize the importance of observing the sensations mindfully and not rushing the process.

- ✓ Adapt the activity for different sensitivity levels, providing alternative methods if needed (e.g., using softer or firmer objects).

Reflection and Journal Activity

Skin Sensation Diary

Keep a diary for a week, noting different skin sensations you experience. Describe the sensations, what caused them, and how they felt. Did you notice any patterns or particularly sensitive areas?

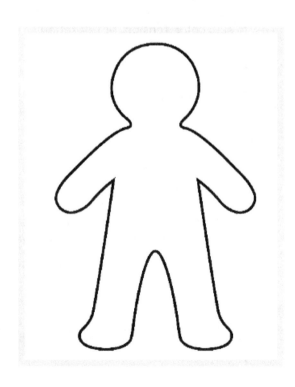

Conclusion

Your skin is an amazing sensory organ that helps you navigate and interact with the world. By understanding and paying attention to the sensations on your skin, you can better protect yourself, enjoy new experiences, and understand your body's needs. Keep exploring and stay curious about the incredible signals your skin sends every day!

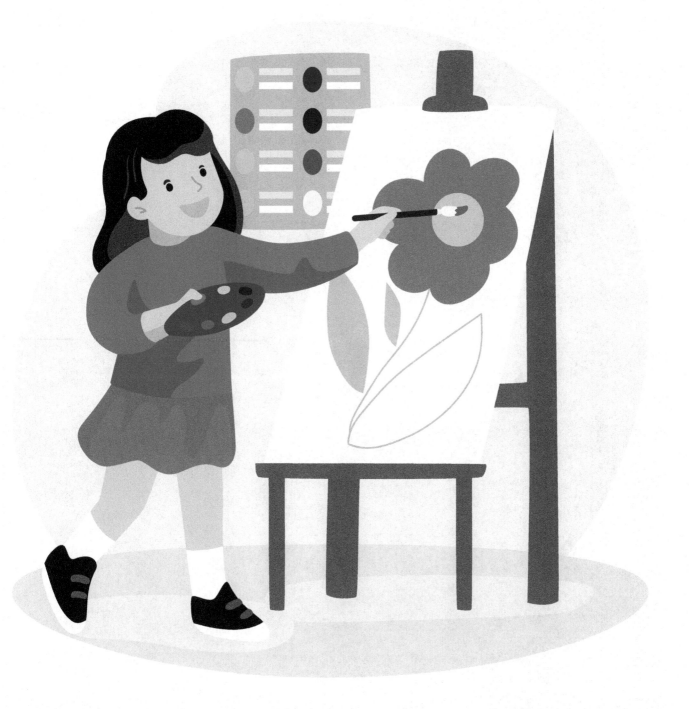

CHAPTER - 5

MUNch MiNdfULLY

A Fun Journey into Mindful Eating

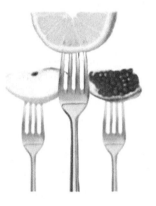

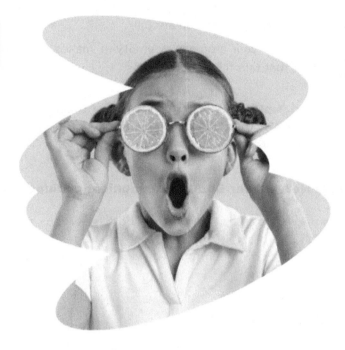

Welcome to the journey to mindful eating! In this chapter, you will complete activities designed to explore taste, thirst, and eating. You will learn about texture and temperature of the food you eat and what happens after digestion. Your body's fuel is important to your health and well-being.

Understanding Hunger

Hunger is like a team effort between your tummy, hormones, and brain. Let's break it down so it is easy to understand:

How Hunger Works:

✓ Hypothalamus : Think of the hypothalamus as the "boss" of hunger in your brain. It helps decide when you are hungry and when you are full.

✓ Ghrelin : When your stomach is empty, it makes a "hunger hormone" called ghrelin. Ghrelin is like a messenger that tells the hypothalamus, "Hey, we need more food!" This makes you feel hungry and ready to eat.

✓ Leptin and Peptide YY : After you eat, your tummy and intestines make "fullness hormones" like leptin and peptide YY. These hormones tell the hypothalamus, "We've had enough food now," so you feel full and stop eating.

The Vagus Nerve: Your Body's Communication Superhighway

The vagus nerve is a crucial part of your body's nervous system, acting like a telephone line that connects your stomach and brain. It sends detailed messages about the activities happening in your stomach and intestines, such as how much food you've eaten and the progress of digestion. Here are some key details about the vagus nerve.

Longest Cranial Nerve

The vagus nerve is the longest of the cranial nerves, extending from the brainstem all the way down to the abdomen. It passes through the neck and chest, branching out to various organs along its path.

Role in Digestion

The vagus nerve controls the muscles in your stomach and intestines, helping to coordinate the movement of food through your digestive tract (peristalsis). It also stimulates the release of digestive enzymes and stomach acids necessary for breaking down food.

✓ Satiety and Hunger Signals : When you've eaten enough, the vagus nerve sends signals to your brain to tell you that you're full, helping to regulate appetite and prevent overeating. But it can also signal hunger when your stomach is empty.

✓ Gut-Brain Axis : The vagus nerve is a critical component of the gut-brain axis, a communication network that links your emotional and cognitive centers in the brain with peripheral intestinal functions. This axis plays a role in emotional well-being and can influence stress levels and mental health.

How It All Works Together

✓ Before Eating : Your stomach is empty, so it makes ghrelin. Ghrelin tells your brain, "I'm hungry!" You feel the urge to eat.

- ✓ While Eating : As you eat, food fills your stomach. The vagus nerve sends messages to your brain saying, "Food is coming in!"
- ✓ After Eating : Your tummy and intestines make leptin and peptide YY. These hormones tell your brain, "We're full now!" You stop feeling hungry and do not want to eat more.

So, when you feel hungry, it is because your stomach and brain are talking to each other, telling you it is time to eat. And when you feel full, it is because they are saying you have had enough food. Your body is good at knowing what it needs!

Understanding Thirst

Thirst happens when our body needs more water to stay balanced. A special part of our brain called the hypothalamus helps control thirst. It works like this:

- ✓ Osmoreceptors : These little sensors in the brain check how much stuff (like salt) is in our blood. If there is too much, they tell us to drink more water.

  Baroreceptors : These sensors keep an eye on our blood pressure. If it drops because we do not have enough blood volume, they tell us to drink more water. When we do not have enough water, our body releases Antidiuretic Hormone (ADH) to help save water.

  Kidneys : They send signals to make us feel thirsty when we need more water. So, when you are feeling thirsty, it is your body's way of saying it needs more water to keep everything working well!

Understanding Thirst

Description: Kids will embark on a fun adventure to become "Hydration Heroes," learning about the importance of drinking water every day through interactive activities, games, and crafts.

Drinking water is important for your body because it helps you stay healthy and strong in many ways! Water keeps your muscles and joints working well, so you can run, jump, and play without getting tired quickly.

It helps you digest your food by breaking it down so your body can use the nutrients to give you energy. Water makes your skin look nice and helps it stay soft and smooth. When you drink enough water, you feel more energetic and can concentrate better at school and during play.

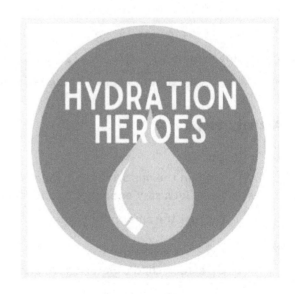

Water is especially important for your brain. Your brain is mostly made of water, so staying hydrated helps it work better. When you drink enough water, you can think more clearly, remember things more easily, and feel more focused. Water helps improve your mood and keeps you from feeling tired or grumpy. It also helps your brain send messages to the rest of your body, so everything works smoothly.

Water helps cool you down when it's hot outside by making you sweat, which keeps your body temperature just right. It also helps flush out any bad stuff from your body, keeping your kidneys healthy. So, remember to drink plenty of water every day to stay happy, healthy, and ready for fun!

Goals

✓ Understand why drinking water is essential for health.

✓ Learn how much water they need to drink daily.

✓ Encourage healthy hydration habits.

Materials Needed

✓ Water bottles

✓ Stickers and markers for decorating water bottles

✓ Hydration chart – make your own or use the one found in the resources section at the back of this book

✓ Measuring cups or water bottles with measurements

✓ Blue construction paper, scissors, glue, and markers for crafts

Daily Water Needs

✓ Children ages 4-8 : about 5 cups (1.2 liters) of water per day

✓ Children ages 9-13 : about 7-8 cups (1.6-1.9 liters) of water per day

✓ Teenagers (ages 14-18) : about 8-11 cups (1.9-2.6 liters) of water per day

✓ Adult women : about 9 cups (2.1 liters) of water per day

✓ Adult men : about 13 cups (3 liters) of water per day

Activity Steps

◉ Introduction

    ✓ Explain the importance of water for the body: it helps with digestion, keeps the skin healthy, and helps kids stay energetic and focused.

    ✓ Discuss the amount of water each child should drink daily.

◉ Water Bottle Decoration

    ✓ Give each child a water bottle and provide stickers, markers, and other decorating materials.

    ✓ Let the kids decorate their water bottles to make them special and encourage them to use them every day.

◉ Hydration Chart

    ✓ Provide each child with a hydration chart. The chart should have spaces for each day of the week and multiple slots per day to track water intake.

    ✓ Explain that each time they drink a glass of water, they can put a sticker or draw a small picture in one of the slots.

Hydration Heroes Chart

DAY	NUMBER OF CUPS (GOAL)	CUP 1	CUP 2	CUP 3	CUP 4	CUP 5	CUP 6	CUP 7	CUP 8
Monday	7-8 cups								
Tuesday	7-8 cups								
Wednesday	7-8 cups								
Thursday	7-8 cups								
Friday	7-8 cups								
Saturday	7-8 cups								
Sunday	7-8 cups								

✅ Hydration Heroes Game

- ✓ Set up a small obstacle course or relay race.
- ✓ At each station, kids need to complete a hydration-related task (e.g., drinking a small cup of water, answering a fun water fact question, or doing a quick water-themed craft).
- ✓ Kids earn "Hydration Hero" badges or stickers after completing each task.

✅ Craft Time - Water Droplet Friends

- ✓ Use blue construction paper to cut out water droplet shapes.
- ✓ Have kids decorate their water droplets with googly eyes, markers, and other craft supplies to create "Water Droplet Friends."
- ✓ Explain that these friends are here to remind them to drink water throughout the day.

✅ Hydration Celebration

- ✓ After completing the activities, gather the kids for a fun celebration.
- ✓ Hand out small prizes or certificates to each "Hydration Hero" for learning about the importance of drinking water.

✅ Discussion and Reflection

- ✓ Gather the kids and ask them to share what they learned about water.
- ✓ Encourage them to take their decorated water bottles and hydration charts home to continue their good habits.

This fun and interactive activity helps kids understand the importance of staying hydrated while engaging them in creative and physical activities.

Taste Sensation Safari

Objective: To help children develop a deeper understanding of different tastes and enhance their sensory awareness through mindful eating.

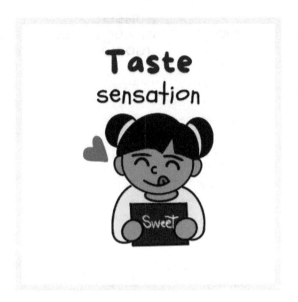

Materials Needed

✓ Small portions of various foods with distinct tastes. See the chart below for more food options.
   - Sweet : apple slices
   - Sour : lemon wedges
   - Salty : pretzels
   - Bitter : dark chocolate
   - Umami : cheese

✓ Blindfolds (optional)

Activity Steps

◔ Introduction

   ✓ Gather the children and explain that they are going on a fun "Taste Sensation Safari" to explore different flavors.

   ✓ Introduce the five basic tastes: sweet, sour, salty, bitter, and umami. Explain each taste briefly:

Types of Taste and Examples of Foods

TYPE OF TASTE	EXAMPLES OF FOODS
Sweet	Apple slices, Strawberries, Honey, Bananas, Mango, Caramel, Peaches, Sweet potatoes
Sour	Lemon wedges, Pickles, Sour candies, Green grapes, Vinegar, Cranberries, Tamarind, Kiwi
Salty	Pretzels, Salted popcorn, Crackers, Olives, Salted nuts, Soy sauce, Potato Chips
Bitter	Dark chocolate, Raw kale, Grapefruit, Brussels sprouts, Coffee, Bitter melon, Arugula, Dandelion greens
Umami	Cheese, Soy sauce, Mushrooms, Cooked tomatoes, Miso soup, Seaweed, Parmesan, Beef broth

◔ Taste Exploration

Step 1: Blind Taste Test (Optional)

- Blindfold the children to help them focus on the taste without being distracted by sight, or simply ask them to close their eyes.

Step 2: Tasting

- Give each child a small portion of one of the foods. Let them take a small bite and really focus on what they are tasting.

Step 3: Describing the Taste

- Encourage the children to describe the taste using words like sweet, tangy, savory, etc. Ask them to also notice how their body feels—do they pucker up with something sour? Do they smile with something sweet?

⊘ Group Sharing

Step 1: Sharing Experiences

- After everyone has tasted the food, gather the children and ask them to share their experiences. What did they taste? How did it make them feel?

Step 2: Comparing Notes

- Compare everyone's reactions and descriptions. Did they all feel the same way about each taste, or were there different reactions? Discuss why some people might taste things differently.

Making It Fun

- ✓ **Safari Theme :** Use a safari theme to make the activity exciting. Pretend you're explorers discovering new flavors in the wild!
- ✓ **Fun Descriptions :** Encourage creative descriptions. For example, "This lemon is as sour as a silly face!" or "This dark chocolate is as bitter as a frown."
- ✓ **Safari Hats and Badges :** Give out little safari hats or badges for participation to make the children feel like real taste adventurers.

By turning the exploration of tastes into a fun and engaging safari adventure, children can enjoy learning about their senses and how they respond to different foods.

Texture Adventure

Objective: To help children become more aware of different food textures and understand how texture can affect their eating experience.

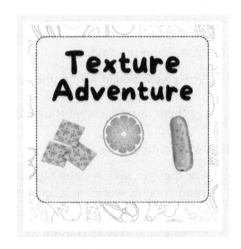

Materials Needed

✓ Small portions of various foods with distinct textures
  - Crunchy : carrot sticks, celery, crackers, pickles
  - Smooth : yogurt, pudding, applesauce
  - Chewy : gummy bears, dried fruit, cheese sticks
  - Soft : bread, cake, marshmallows
  - Juicy : watermelon, grapes, oranges
✓ Blindfolds (optional)
✓ Small bags or containers for each type of food
✓ Stickers and markers for decorating the bags

Activity Steps

◉ Introduction
  ✓ Gather the children and explain that they are going on a "Texture Treasure Hunt" to discover and explore different food textures.
  ✓ Introduce the concept of texture and how it influences our eating experience. Explain how paying attention to texture can make eating more enjoyable and mindful.
  ✓ Use fun analogies, such as
    - "Crunchy foods are like walking on crunchy leaves in the fall."
    - "Smooth foods are like a silky blanket."
    - "Chewy foods are like chewing bubble gum."
    - "Soft foods are like a fluffy pillow."
    - "Juicy foods are like biting into a water balloon!"

◉ Texture Exploration

Step 1: Blind Texture Test (Optional)

- Blindfold the children to enhance their focus on texture without being distracted by sight, or simply ask them to close their eyes.

Step 2: Feeling the Texture

- Provide each child with a small portion of one of the foods. Ask them to feel the food with their hands before tasting it.
- Let them describe what they feel using words like bumpy, smooth, squishy, or hard.

Step 3: Tasting and Describing

- Ask them to take a small bite and focus on the texture. Encourage children to describe the texture using specific words (e.g., crunchy, smooth, chewy).
- Make it fun by using playful descriptions, like "This cracker is as crunchy as stepping on dry leaves!" or "This yogurt is as smooth as a slide!"

✐ Group Sharing

    Step 1: Sharing Experiences

- After exploring each texture, gather the children and ask them to share their experiences and descriptions with the group.
- Use a "Texture Treasure Map" where each child can place a sticker representing the texture they explored.

    Step 2: Comparing Notes

- Compare the different reactions and descriptions, discussing any similarities or differences.
- Celebrate everyone's discoveries by giving them "Texture Explorer" badges.

Making It Fun

✓   **Decorating Bags/Containers** : Let children decorate the bags or containers holding each type of food with stickers and markers. They can draw pictures that represent the texture (e.g., bumpy lines for crunchy, wavy lines for smooth).

✓   **Texture Treasure Map** : Create a large map on a poster board where children can place stickers representing each texture they discover. For example, place a carrot sticker on the "Crunchy" section and a yogurt sticker on the "Smooth" section.

✓   **Treasure Hunt Clues** : Give out fun clues or riddles for each food texture. For example, "Find the food that's as crunchy as stepping on dry leaves!" or "Look for the treat that's as smooth as a slide!"

✓   **Explorer Badges** : Make "Texture Explorer" badges for each child to wear during the activity. They can earn different badges for discovering different textures.

✓   **Story Time** : After the activity, gather the children for a story about a brave explorer who discovers new textures in a magical food forest. This can reinforce the fun and learning experience.

Fun food analogies to use during this activity.

- **Crispy** : This potato chip is as crispy as autumn leaves under your feet.

- **Silky** : This yogurt is as silky as sliding down a slide covered in super soft blankets.

- **Bouncy** : These jellybeans are as bouncy as a rubber ball dropped from high up.

- **Fluffy** : This pancake is as fluffy as a kitten's fur.

- **Flavor Explosion** : This grape is as bursting with flavor as a freshly opened can of soda.

- **Crackling** : This popcorn is as crackling as a campfire on a starry night.

- **Velvety** : This chocolate mousse is as smooth as petting a velvety bunny.

- **Elastic** : This licorice is as elastic as a rubber band pulled and stretched.

- **Pillow-like** : This cotton candy is as pillow-like as a cloud in the sky.

- **Drippy** : This peach is so juicy, it's like taking a big sip of the sweetest, yummiest juice ever.

By making the Texture Treasure Hunt engaging and playful, children will have a fun time learning about different food textures and how they affect their eating experience.

Environment Eating Adventure

Objective: To help children understand how their eating environment can affect their eating experience and emotions.

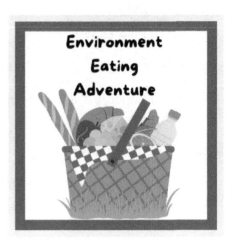

Materials Needed

✓ Different eating environments (e.g., a quiet space, a noisy space, an outdoor area, a brightly lit area)

✓ Small portions of the same food for each environment

✓ Fun props to set the scene (e.g., blankets for a picnic, lamps for lighting)

✓ Notebooks or paper for drawing and writing

Activity Steps

☑ Introduction

    ✓ Gather the children and explain that they are going on an "Environment Eating Adventure" to discover how different surroundings can change the way they experience food.

    ✓ Discuss how the environment can influence our eating experience and emotions. For example, a quiet room might make eating feel calm, while a noisy room might make it harder to concentrate on the taste.

    ✓ Explain the importance of being aware of our surroundings when eating and how it can help us enjoy our food more.

☑ Environment Exploration

Step 1: Eating in Different Environments

- Guide the children to various eating environments set up around the area (e.g., a quiet corner with pillows, a noisy room with music playing, an outdoor picnic area, a brightly lit room).

- Provide each child with the same portion of food in each environment. Make the setup fun with props like picnic blankets, lamps, or music players.

Step 2: Observing and Tasting

- Ask the children to take a bite of the food in each environment and focus on how it tastes and how they feel.

- Encourage them to notice any changes in taste, enjoyment, and their mood.

☑ Group Sharing

Step 1: Sharing Experiences

- After exploring each environment, gather the children and ask them to share their experiences. Use questions like:

- "How did the food taste in the quiet room?"

- "Did the noisy room change how you felt about the food?"

- "What was it like eating outside?"

- "Did the bright lights make any difference?"

Step 2: Comparing Notes

- Compare the different reactions and descriptions. Discuss any similarities or differences in how they experienced the food in each environment.

Making It Extra Fun

✓ Environment Themes : Create themed environments to make the adventure more exciting. For example:

- Quiet Space : Cozy reading nook with pillows and soft music.

- Noisy Space : Dance party room with upbeat music and colorful lights.

- Outdoor Area : Picnic blanket with nature sounds playing.

- Brightly Lit Area : Room with bright lamps and cheerful decorations.

✓ Explorer Badges : Give out "Environment Explorer" badges to each child for participating in the adventure.

✓ Drawing and Writing : Provide notebooks or paper for the children to draw or write about their experiences in each environment. Encourage them to illustrate how the food looked and felt in different settings.

✓ Mystery Food : Add an element of surprise by including a "mystery food" in each environment for the children to taste and guess.

Example Questions for Group Sharing:

✓ "Which environment was your favorite for eating? Why?"

✓ "Did any environment make the food taste better or worse?"

✓ "How did you feel in each environment? Relaxed, excited, distracted?"

✓ "Did the environment remind you of any special memories or places?"

By turning the Environment Eating Adventure into a fun and engaging activity, children will have a memorable experience learning about how their surroundings can affect their eating experience and emotions.

✓ Under the Sea Adventure

- Setup : Decorate the eating area with blue and green streamers to represent water. Use fish cutouts, seashells, and ocean-themed tablecloths. Play soft ocean sounds in the background.

- Props : Provide paper fish hats or masks for the children to wear.

- Food : Serve food on blue plates and ask children to imagine they are mermaids or underwater explorers.

- ✓ Space Picnic
  - Setup : Create a space-themed area with black tablecloths, glow-in-the-dark stars, and planet cutouts. Use silver foil to cover surfaces for a futuristic look. Play space sounds or soft electronic music.
  - Props : Give each child a "space helmet" made from aluminum foil or paper plates.
  - Food : Serve food in small containers labeled as "space food" and encourage children to pretend they are astronauts on a mission.

- ✓ Jungle Safari
  - Setup : Decorate with green and brown streamers, fake plants, and animal prints. Use animal figurines and play jungle sounds like birds chirping and leaves rustling.
  - Props : Provide safari hats and binoculars (made from toilet paper rolls) for the children.
  - Food : Serve food on leaf-shaped plates or banana leaves. Encourage children to imagine they are explorers in a jungle.

- ✓ Royal Feast
  - Setup : Create a royal dining area with elegant tablecloths, pretend gold utensils, and "goblets" (plastic cups). Use crowns and tiaras as decorations. Play classical music in the background.
  - Props : Give each child a crown or tiara to wear during the feast.
  - Food : Serve food on fancy-looking plates and encourage children to pretend they are kings, queens, princes, or princesses enjoying a royal banquet.

- ✓ Camping Trip
  - Setup : Set up a camping area with a small tent or makeshift tent using blankets. Use picnic blankets, lanterns, and pretend campfires (made from paper or LED lights). Play nature sounds like crickets and crackling campfires.
  - Props : Provide each child with a "camping badge" and small backpacks.
  - Food : Serve food on tin plates or bowls and encourage children to imagine they are campers eating under the stars.

- ✓ Fairy Garden
  - Setup : Decorate with twinkling fairy lights, flower garlands, and small fairy figurines. Use soft pastel colors for tablecloths and play gentle harp music.
  - Props : Provide fairy wings or wands for the children.
  - Food : Serve food on flower-shaped plates and encourage children to imagine they are fairies in a magical garden.

- ✓ Pirate Island
  - Setup : Decorate with pirate flags, treasure chests, and maps. Use sand (or sand-colored fabric) and seashells for added effect. Play pirate-themed music or ocean waves.
  - Props : Swords and eye patches.
  - Food : Serve food in small treasure chests or on pirate-themed plates. Encourage children to imagine they are pirates searching for treasure.

By incorporating these creative and immersive themes, you can make the Environment Eating Adventure even more exciting and memorable for the children, enhancing their learning experience about interoception and the impact of different environments on their eating habits.

Thirsty Explorers Adventure

Objective : To help children understand and recognize the signals of thirst in their bodies and learn about interoception through fun, interactive activities.

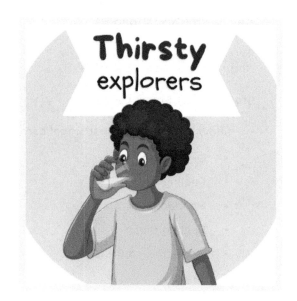

Materials Needed

✓ Small water bottles or cups of water for each child

✓ A variety of activities that make children slightly active (e.g., jumping jacks, running in place, dancing)

✓ Thirst signal cards (illustrations or descriptions of signs of thirst like dry mouth, feeling tired, headache, etc.)

✓ Stickers or stamps for marking progress (optional)

✓ Notebooks or paper for drawing and writing reflections

Thirst Signals

✓ Dry Mouth : Your mouth feels dry and sticky.

✓ Feeling Tired : You start to feel sleepy or less energetic.

✓ Headache : You get a headache that might feel like a dull ache.

✓ Feeling Dizzy : You feel lightheaded or dizzy.

✓ Dark-Colored Urine : Your pee is a darker color than usual.

✓ Dry Skin : Your skin feels dry or rough.

✓ Feeling Thirsty : You have a strong desire to drink something.

✓ Muscle Cramps : Your muscles feel tight or cramp up.

✓ Lack of Focus : You find it hard to concentrate or pay attention.

✓ Dry Eyes : Your eyes feel dry or irritated.

✓ Rapid Heartbeat : Your heart feels like it is beating faster than usual.

✓ Decreased Urination : You are not going to the bathroom as often.

Activity Steps

✓ Introduction

✓ Gather the children and explain that they are going to become "Thirsty Explorers" to learn how their bodies tell them when they need water.

✓ Discuss why it is important to recognize when they are thirsty and how drinking water helps their bodies stay healthy and strong.

✓ Understanding Thirst Signals

Step 1: Thirst Signal Cards

- Show the children thirst signal cards and explain each sign of thirst, such as:
    - Dry mouth
    - Feeling tired
    - Headache
    - Feeling dizzy
    - Dark-colored urine
    - Dry skin
    - Feeling thirsty
    - Muscle cramps
    - Lack of focus
    - Dry eyes
    - Rapid heartbeat
    - Decreased urination
- Make it interactive by asking the children to mimic or act out each signal.

✓ Thirsty Explorers Activities

Step 1: Active Exploration

- Guide the children through a series of light physical activities to make them slightly active. Activities can include:
    - Jumping jacks
    - Running in place
    - Dancing to fun music
    - A mini obstacle course
- Keep the activities fun and engaging, ensuring they get a little bit thirsty.

Recognizing Thirst

Step 1: Checking for Thirst Signals

- After the physical activities, gather the children and ask them how they feel. Encourage them to check for any thirst signals they learned about.
- Use questions like:
    - "Is your mouth feeling dry?"
    - "Do you feel a little tired or dizzy?"
    - "Do you have a slight headache?"
    - "Are your eyes feeling dry?"
    - "Do your muscles feel tight?"
    - "Is your heart beating faster than usual?"
- Discuss their observations and reinforce the idea that these signals mean their body needs water.

Drinking Water

Step 1: Hydration Time

- Provide each child with a small water bottle or cup of water. Ask them to take a few sips and pay attention to how their body feels as they drink.
- Encourage them to notice any changes, such as their mouth feeling less dry or having more energy.

Reflection and Sharing

Step 1: Group Sharing

- After drinking water, gather the children and ask them to share their experiences. Use questions like:
    - "How did you feel before and after drinking water?"
    - "What signals did your body give you to tell you that you were thirsty?"
    - "How does drinking water help you feel better?"

Step 2: Drawing and Writing Reflections

- Provide notebooks or paper for the children to draw or write about their "Thirsty Explorers" adventure. Encourage them to illustrate how they felt before and after drinking water.

Celebration

Step 1: Group Celebration

- Celebrate their success with a group cheer or a fun game. Reinforce the idea that they have learned valuable skills about listening to their bodies' thirst signals.

Additional Fun Elements

✓   Theme the Adventure : Use themes like "Desert Trek" or "Jungle Expedition" to make the activities more exciting.

✓   Interactive Storytelling : Create a story around the adventure, such as exploring a desert and needing to find water to stay hydrated.

✓   Water Fun : Include fun water-related activities, like a mini water balloon toss or a splash area, to reinforce the importance of staying hydrated.

By making the Thirsty Explorers Adventure engaging and interactive, children will have a fun time learning about interoception and how to recognize their body's signals for thirst.

My Food and Drink Fuel Journal

Objective : To help children become more aware of their eating and drinking habits by keeping a journal for a week, enhancing their understanding of interoception, and promoting healthy choices.

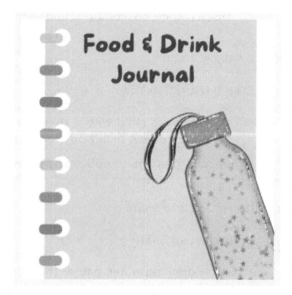

Goals

✓   Increase awareness of eating habits

✓   Understand the connection between food and emotions

✓   Promote mindful eating

✓   Identify patterns in food choices and their effects on the body

✓   Encourage self-reflection and healthier eating habits

Materials Needed

✓   Blank notebooks or printed journal pages

✓   Markers, crayons, and stickers for decorating the journals

✓   Sample journal pages with prompts

✓   Example entries for guidance

✓   A calendar or planner (optional)

✓   Small rewards or certificates for completion (optional)

Activity Steps

✓ Set Up Your Fuel Diary

✓ Create a Fuel Diary template in a notebook or print out a pre-made template.

✓ Decorate your diary with stickers, drawings, or colorful markers to make it personal and fun.

✓ When children create their own journal, they feel more empowered to engage and participate.

✓ Track Your Intake

✓ For one week, write down everything you eat and drink in your Fuel Diary.

✓ Include the time of day for each entry to help identify any patterns.

✓ Reflect on Your Food

✓ In the third column, write down your thoughts about the food or drink. Consider aspects like taste, texture, and satisfaction.

✓ Ask yourself questions like: Did I enjoy this food? Was it satisfying? Did it remind me of anything?

✓ Observe Your Feelings

✓ In the fourth column, note how you feel after eating or drinking. Consider physical and emotional responses.

✓ Ask yourself questions like: Do I feel energized or tired? Am I satisfied or still hungry? How is my mood?

✓ Daily Review

✓ At the end of each day, review your Fuel Diary entries. Look for patterns in your eating habits and how different foods make you feel.

✓ Reflect on whether certain foods or drinks consistently make you feel good or not.

✓ Weekly Reflection

✓ At the end of the week, take some time to review your entire Fuel Diary.

✓ Write a summary of your observations, such as which foods made you feel the best and which ones did not.

✓ Consider any changes you might want to make to your eating habits based on your reflections.

Example Entries

TIME	TYPE OF FOOD/ DRINK	WHAT DID I THINK ABOUT THE FOOD?	HOW I FEEL AFTER EATING
7:30 AM	Oatmeal with blueberries	It was warm and sweet. I liked the berries.	Full and ready to play
10:00 AM	Banana	It was soft and sweet. Easy to eat.	Energized
12:00 PM	Peanut butter & jelly sandwich	It was sticky and salty. Stuck to top of my mouth	Relaxed, happy and focused
3:00 PM	Yogurt	It was creamy and tangy. Ate with my favorite spoon	Happy tummy
6:00 PM	Chicken nuggets and beans	It was savory and yummy	Sleepy but ready to go outside
8:00 PM	Ice Cream	Cold and wet. My tongue was numb.	Silly and cold

Additional Activities

- Daily Tracking

Step 1: Encouraging Daily Entries

- Encourage the children to make entries in their journals every day for a week. Remind them to note everything they eat and drink and how they feel.

Step 2: Set Reminders

- If possible, set daily reminders for the children to fill out their journals. This can be a fun group activity at the end of each day.

- Reflection and Sharing

Step 1: Group Sharing

- At the end of the week, gather the children to share their journal experiences. Use questions like:
  - "What did you notice about what you ate and drank this week?"
  - "Did you feel differently after eating certain foods or drinking more water?"
  - "What was your favorite meal or snack?"

Step 2: Drawing and Writing Reflections

- Provide additional pages for the children to draw or write about their week-long food and drink adventure. Encourage them to illustrate their favorite meal or how they felt throughout the week.

- Celebration

  ### Step 1: Completion Certificates

  - Give each child a small reward or certificate for completing their Fuel Journal.

  ### Step 2: Group Celebration

  - Celebrate their success with a fun group activity, like a healthy snack party or a game. Reinforce the idea that they have learned valuable skills about paying attention to what they eat and drink.

Additional Fun Elements

✓ Healthy Eating Challenges : Introduce fun challenges for the week, such as trying a new fruit or vegetable each day or drinking a certain number of glasses of water.

✓ Interactive Storytelling : Create a story about a character who learns about healthy eating and drinking habits, and how it helps them feel better.

✓ Recipe Sharing : Have a session where children can share their favorite healthy recipes or snacks with the group.

Hydration Detective : Learning About Urine Colors and Hydration

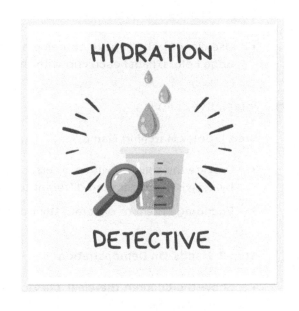

Objective : To help children understand how the color of their urine relates to their hydration levels and learn about interoception in a fun and engaging way.

Materials Needed

✓ Clear plastic cups or containers

✓ Food coloring (yellow, light yellow, dark yellow, amber, and brown)

✓ Water

✓ Posters or signs with information about urine color and hydration

✓ Markers, crayons, and stickers for decorating

✓ Hydration chart printouts (showing different urine colors and what they mean)

✓ Healthy snacks and drinks (e.g., water, fruits, juice)

✓ Notebooks or paper for reflections

Activity Steps

☑ Introduction

✓ Gather the children and explain that they will be learning about hydration and how to tell if they need more water by looking at the color of their urine.

✓ Discuss why staying hydrated is important for their health, energy levels, and overall well-being.

☑ Understanding Urine Colors

Step 1: Creating a Hydration Chart

- Show the children a hydration chart with different urine colors and explain what each color means:
    - Clear or Very Light Yellow : **Very well-hydrated**
    - Light Yellow : **Hydrated**
    - Yellow : **Slightly dehydrated**
    - Dark Yellow : **Dehydrated, need to drink more water**
    - Amber or Honey : **Very dehydrated, need to drink water immediately**
    - Brown : **Severely dehydrated, need to drink water immediately and possibly seek medical help**
    - Pink or Red : **Could be due to certain foods or a sign of blood in the urine; consult a doctor**
    - Blue or Green : **Could be due to certain foods or medications; consult a doctor**

Step 2: Making the Hydration Chart

- Use clear plastic cups or containers filled with water and food coloring to create samples of different urine colors. Label each cup with the corresponding hydration level.

☑ Interactive Learning

Step 1: Color Matching Game

- Provide the children with markers, crayons, and stickers. Ask them to create their own hydration chart by drawing and coloring different urine colors and writing what each color means next to it.

- Encourage them to decorate their charts and make them colorful and fun.

Step 2: Hands-On Demonstration

- Show the children the clear plastic cups with colored water. Ask them to match each color to the hydration level on the chart.

- Discuss how they can use this information to check their own hydration levels by looking at the color of their urine.

- ☑ Hydration Station

Step 1: Serving Drinks and Snacks

- Set up a hydration station with healthy drinks like water, fruit-infused water, and juice, along with hydrating snacks like fruits and vegetables.
- Encourage the children to choose drinks and snacks that help keep them hydrated.

Step 2: Drinking Water and Noticing Changes

- Ask the children to drink a cup of water and pay attention to how their bodies feel before and after drinking. Use prompts like:
  - "How does your mouth feel after drinking water?"
  - "Do you feel more refreshed?"

- ☑ Reflection and Sharing

Step 1: Group Sharing

- After the hydration station, gather the children and ask them to share their experiences. Use questions like:
  - "What did you learn about the color of your urine and hydration?"
  - "How can you tell if you need to drink more water?"
  - "What was your favorite part of the activity?"

Step 2: Drawing and Writing Reflections

- Provide notebooks or paper for the children to draw or write about their "Hydration Detective" adventure. Encourage them to illustrate their hydration chart and what they learned about staying hydrated.

- ☑ Celebration

Step 1: Group Celebration

- Celebrate their success with a group cheer or a fun game. Reinforce the idea that they have learned valuable skills about checking their hydration levels and the importance of drinking enough water.

Additional Fun Elements

✓ Themed Hydration Station:Use themes like "Under the Sea" or "Jungle Adventure" to make the hydration station more exciting.

✓ Desert Station: Talk about desert biome and how a cactus does not need frequent rain because it can store water. Look up animals and average rain.

✓ Interactive Storytelling: Create a story about a character who learns the importance of staying hydrated and how to check their urine color.

✓ Hydration Challenges: Introduce fun challenges, such as drinking a certain number of cups of water each day or trying different hydrating fruits.

By making the Hydration Detective activity engaging and interactive, children will have a fun time learning about interoception and the importance of staying hydrated by understanding the color of their urine.

Poop Patrol: Exploring the World of Stool

Objective : To help children understand the different types of stool using the Bristol Stool Chart and a fun, hands-on activity with brown dough.

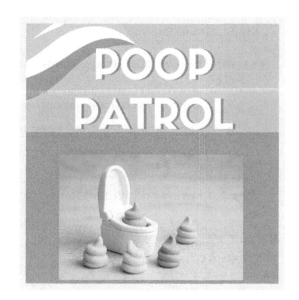

Materials Needed

✓ Brown dough or clay (enough for each child to create multiple types of stools)

✓ Bristol Stool Chart printouts (with child-friendly descriptions and pictures)

✓ Disposable gloves (optional)

✓ Plastic mats or trays for working with the dough

✓ Markers, crayons, and stickers for decorating the charts

✓ Notebooks or paper for reflections

✓ Healthy snacks and drinks (optional)

IMPORTANT NOTE:
Avoid this activity if your child/student engages in fecal smearing, known as Scatolia. If your child shows unusual interest in stool, consult your physician. Causes could be sensory-related, parasitic infection, constipation, PICA, anxiety, or other medical reasons.

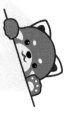

Activity Steps

✓ Introduction

✓ Gather the children and explain that they will be learning about different types of stool and what they can tell us about our digestion.

✓ Use the Bristol Stool Chart to introduce the seven types of stool, explaining in simple terms what each type means for their health.

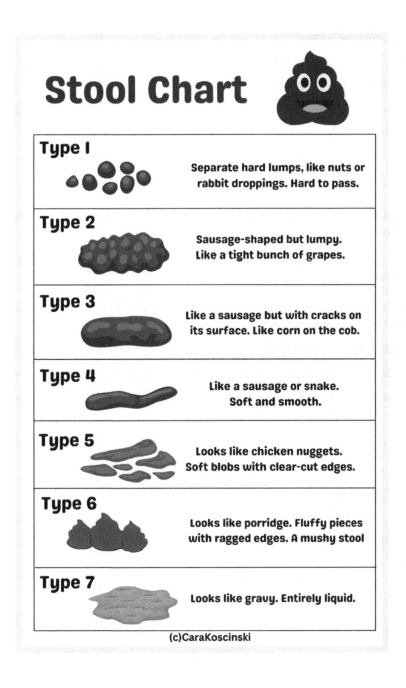

Stool Chart

Type 1
Separate hard lumps, like nuts or rabbit droppings. Hard to pass.

Type 2
Sausage-shaped but lumpy. Like a tight bunch of grapes.

Type 3
Like a sausage but with cracks on its surface. Like corn on the cob.

Type 4
Like a sausage or snake. Soft and smooth.

Type 5
Looks like chicken nuggets. Soft blobs with clear-cut edges.

Type 6
Looks like porridge. Fluffy pieces with ragged edges. A mushy stool

Type 7
Looks like gravy. Entirely liquid.

(c)CaraKoscinski

Understanding the Bristol Stool Chart

Step 1: Introducing the Chart

- Show the children a Bristol Stool Chart with child-friendly descriptions and pictures:
    - Type 1: Separate hard lumps, like nuts (hard to pass) – Could mean constipation.
    - Type 2: Sausage-shaped but lumpy – Slightly constipated.
    - Type 3: Like a sausage but with cracks on its surface – Normal.
    - Type 4: Like a sausage or snake, smooth and soft – Normal.
    - Type 5: Soft blobs with clear-cut edges (easy to pass) – Lacking fiber.
    - Type 6: Fluffy pieces with ragged edges, a mushy stool – Mild diarrhea.
    - Type 7: Watery, no solid pieces, entirely liquid – Diarrhea.
- Discuss how different types of stools can indicate how their digestive system is working.

Poop Patrol: Creating Different Types of Stool

Step 1: Preparing the Dough

- Give each child a portion of brown dough or clay. Explain that they will be making different types of stools based on the Bristol Stool Chart.

Step 2: Creating the Stools

- Use plastic mats or trays for working with the dough. Ask the children to use the dough to create each type of stool according to the chart.
- Provide disposable gloves if preferred.
- Encourage them to make the shapes and textures as close as possible to the descriptions:
    - Separate hard lumps for Type 1.
    - Sausage-shaped but lumpy for Type 2.
    - Sausage-shaped with cracks for Type 3.
    - Smooth and soft sausage or snake for Type 4.
    - Soft blobs for Type 5.
    - Fluffy, mushy pieces for Type 6.
    - Watery texture for Type 7 (use more imagination and less dough for this).

✓ Interactive Learning

Step 1: Discussing the Creations

- After creating the different types of stools, gather the children and discuss what they made. Use questions like:
  - "What does Type 1 stool look and feel like?"
  - "How did you make Type 4 stool smooth and soft?"
  - "Why is it important to know about Type 7 stool?"

Step 2: Matching with the Chart

- Ask the children to match their dough creations to the pictures on the Bristol Stool Chart. Discuss any differences and similarities they notice.

✓ Reflection and Sharing

Step 1: Group Sharing

- Gather the children and ask them to share their experiences. Use questions like:
  - "What did you learn about different types of stool?"
  - "How can you tell if your stool is healthy?"
  - "What was your favorite part of the activity?"

Step 2: Drawing and Writing Reflections

- Provide notebooks or paper for the children to draw or write about their "Poop Patrol" adventure. Encourage them to illustrate their favorite stool type and what they learned about their digestive health.

✓ Celebration

Step 1: Group Celebration

- Celebrate their success with a group cheer or a fun game. Reinforce the idea that they have learned valuable skills about recognizing different types of stool and their importance for health.

Step 2: Healthy Snacks (Optional)

- Provide healthy snacks and drinks to emphasize the importance of a balanced diet for good digestive health.

Additional Fun Elements

✓ Themed Dough Kits : Provide dough kits with different colors and textures to make the activity more engaging.

✓ Interactive Storytelling : Create a story about a character who goes on a "Poop Patrol" adventure to learn about healthy digestion.

By making the Poop Patrol activity engaging and interactive, children will have a fun time learning about interoception and the importance of recognizing different types of stool for their digestive health.

Temperature Taste Test: Exploring Warm and Cold Foods and Drinks

Objective : To help children understand how different temperatures of food and drinks feel in their mouths and learn about interoception through a fun, hands-on activity.

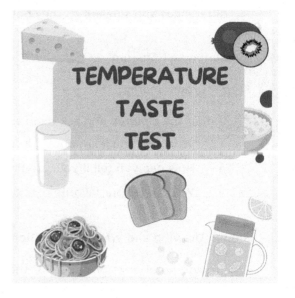

Examples of Hot Foods

✓ Soup : Warm chicken or vegetable soup.

✓ Hot Chocolate : A warm, comforting cup of hot chocolate.

✓ Warm Fruit Slices : Apple slices warmed in the microwave or oven.

✓ Grilled Cheese Sandwich : A freshly made grilled cheese sandwich.

✓ Mashed Potatoes : Warm, creamy mashed potatoes.

✓ Hot Cereal : A bowl of hot oatmeal or grits.

✓ Bread : Warm slices of freshly baked bread or toast.

✓ Hot Pasta : A small serving of warm pasta or mac and cheese.

✓ Steamed Vegetables : Warm, steamed broccoli, corn, or carrots.

✓ Warmed Food of Child's Preference : A slice of pizza, chicken nuggets, burger.

Examples of Cold Foods

✓ Ice Cream: A scoop of cold ice cream or frozen yogurt.

✓ Water: A glass of cold water with ice cubes or shaved ice.

✓ Cold Fruit Slices: Apple slices, peaches, watermelon served cold from the refrigerator.

✓ Cheese: Cold cheese cubes or slices.

✓ Yogurt: A cup of cold yogurt.

✓ Cold Pasta Salad : A small serving of cold pasta salad.

✓ Smoothie : A cold fruit smoothie.

✓ Fruit Salad : A bowl of cold fruit salad.

✓ Popsicles : Cold, refreshing popsicles.

✓ Cold Milk : A glass of cold milk.

Activity Steps (with Examples):

✅ Introduction

Gather the children and explain that they will be learning about how different temperatures of food and drinks feel in their mouths.

Discuss the importance of paying attention to these sensations and how it helps them enjoy and understand their food better.

✅ Setting Up the Taste Test

Step 1: Preparing the Foods and Drinks

- Prepare small portions of various warm and cold foods and drinks. Use small cups and bowls for serving.

Step 2: Decorating the Area

- Set up a table with warm and cold food and drinks. Use decorations like tablecloths, posters, and signs to make the area inviting and fun.
- Provide markers, crayons, and stickers for the children to decorate their own "Temperature Taste Test" placemats.

✅ Temperature Taste Test

Step 1: Trying Hot Foods and Drinks

- Start with hot foods and drinks. Serve each child a small portion and ask them to taste it.
- Encourage them to pay attention to how the hot food or drink feels in their mouth. Use prompts like:
    - "How does the hot chocolate feel on your tongue?"
    - "Does the warm soup make you feel cozy?"
- Ask them to describe the sensation using words like "warm," "hot," "comforting," or "soothing."

Step 2: Trying Cold Foods and Drinks

- Move on to cold foods and drinks. Serve each child a small portion and ask them to taste it.

- Encourage them to pay attention to how the cold food or drink feels in their mouth. Use prompts like:

  - "How does the ice cream feel on your tongue?"

  - "Does the ice water make you feel refreshed?"

- Ask them to describe the sensation using words like "cold," "cool," "refreshing," or "chilly."

Interactive Learning

Step 1: Discussing Sensations

- After tasting the hot and cold foods and drinks, gather the children and discuss their experiences. Use questions like:

  - "Which hot food or drink was your favorite?"

  - "How did the cold foods and drinks make you feel?"

  - "Did you notice any differences in how your mouth felt with hot versus cold items?"

Step 2: Matching Sensations to Foods

- Provide posters or charts with pictures of the foods and drinks they tasted. Ask the children to match the sensations they felt to the pictures.

- Discuss any differences and similarities they noticed.

Reflection and Sharing

Step 1: Group Sharing

- Gather the children and ask them to share their experiences. Use questions like:

  - "What did you learn about how hot and cold foods and drinks feel in your mouth?"

  - "How can you tell if something is too hot or too cold to eat or drink?"

  - "What was your favorite part of the activity?"

Step 2: Drawing and Writing Reflections

- Provide notebooks or paper for the children to draw or write about their "Temperature Taste Test" adventure. Encourage them to illustrate their favorite hot and cold foods and how they felt while tasting them.

Additional Fun Elements

✓ Themed Taste Test: Use themes like "Winter Wonderland" for cold items and "Cozy Campfire" for hot items to make the activity more exciting.

✓ Interactive Storytelling: Create a story about a character who goes on a taste test adventure to learn about hot and cold foods and drinks.

✓ Temperature Challenges: Introduce fun challenges, such as guessing the temperature of different foods and drinks or finding their favorite hot and cold combinations.

By making the Temperature Taste Test engaging and interactive, children will have a fun time learning about interoception and the importance of recognizing how different temperatures of food and drinks feel in their mouths.

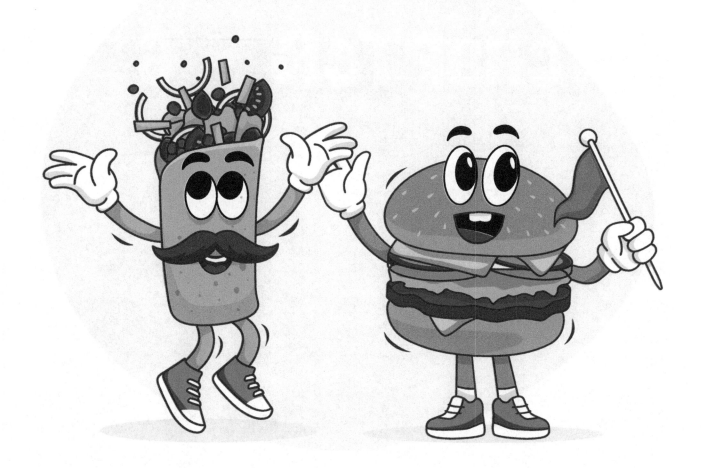

CHAPTER - 6

POWER UP YOUR CALM

Breathing Activities

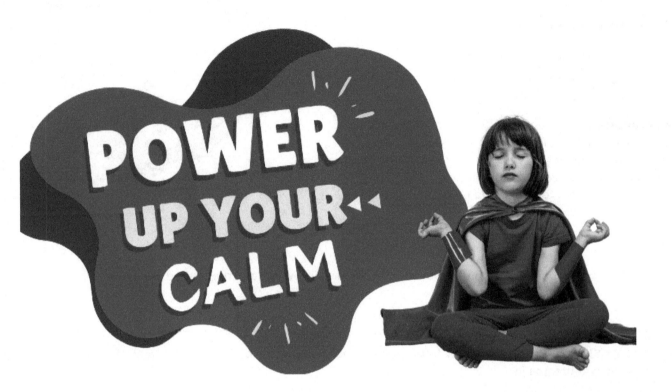

Introduction

Welcome to Chapter 6 of your interoception adventure! In this chapter, we are going to learn how to power up your calm using different breathing activities. Breathing is not just about taking in air; it is a superpower that can help you feel relaxed, focused, and calm. When you practice breathing exercises, you help your body and mind to relax, increase the oxygen supply to your brain, and improve your overall well-being. Get ready to discover how powerful your breath can be.

NOTE: While practicing breathing exercises, it is essential to listen to your body and be mindful of how you feel. If you start to feel dizzy, lightheaded, or uncomfortable, stop the exercise and take a break. Always practice these exercises in a safe and comfortable environment, and if you have any medical conditions or concerns, consult with a healthcare professional before starting new breathing activities.

Stuffed Friend Breaths

Objective : To practice deep breathing and understand how it helps calm the body and mind.

Materials Needed

- A comfortable spot to sit or lie down
- A stuffed animal or small pillow

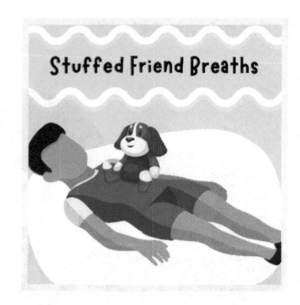

Explanation : Deep breathing, or diaphragmatic breathing, helps activate your body's relaxation response. It can slow your heart rate, lower blood pressure, and increase the amount of oxygen in your blood, making you feel calm and relaxed.

Steps

- **Get Comfortable:** Find a comfortable spot to sit or lie down. Place the stuffed animal or pillow on your belly.
  - Tip : Choose a favorite stuffed animal to make this activity even more enjoyable.

- **Inhale Slowly:** Breathe in slowly through your nose, filling your belly with air. Watch the stuffed animal rise as you breathe in.
  - Visualization : Imagine you are filling up a balloon in your belly.

- **Exhale Slowly:** Breathe out slowly through your mouth, letting your belly fall. Watch the stuffed animal go down as you breathe out.
  - Visualization: Picture the balloon gently deflating.

- **Repeat:** Do this for 5-10 breaths, paying attention to the rise and fall of your stuffed animal. Notice how calm and relaxed you start to feel.
  - Challenge : Try to make each breath last a little longer than the previous one.

Extension Activities

- **Story Time Breaths:** After the breathing exercise, have your child tell a short story about their stuffed animal's adventure during the rise and fall of their breaths.
- **Breathing Buddies:** Pair up with a friend or family member and do the breathing exercise together, each with their own stuffed animal. Compare how high each stuffed animal rises.

Reflection Questions

✓   How did you feel before and after the breathing exercise?

✓   Did you notice any changes in how your body felt?

✓   What other times might deep breathing help you feel calm?

Count Your Breath

Objective : To learn how to control the length of your breath and create a calming rhythm.

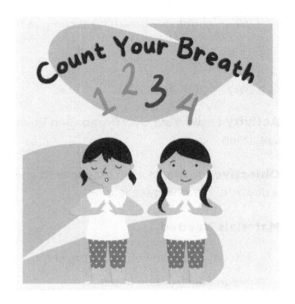

Materials Needed

✓   A quiet place to sit

Explanation : Controlling your breath by counting helps regulate your breathing pattern. This can help you focus, reduce stress, and bring more oxygen to your brain, enhancing your sense of calm and relaxation.

Steps

✅   Inhale and Count : Breathe in slowly through your nose while counting to 4 in your head.
   •   Tip : Imagine your lungs filling up like a balloon as you count.

✅   Hold: Hold your breath for a count of 4.
   •   Tip : Think of this pause as giving your body a moment to soak in all the fresh air.

✅   Exhale and Count: Breathe out slowly through your mouth while counting to 4.
   •   Tip : Picture gently blowing out a candle as you exhale.

✅   Hold :   Hold your breath for a count of 4.
   •   Tip : This pause is like a little rest for your body before starting the next breath.

✅   Repeat :   Continue this pattern for a few minutes. Try to keep the counts even and notice how your body feels more relaxed with each breath.
   •   Challenge : Gradually increase the count to 5 or 6 if you feel comfortable.

Extension Activities

✓   Counting Fun : Use your fingers to count as you breathe in and out, making it easier to keep track.

✓   Visual Aid : Imagine a calm scene, like waves gently rolling in and out, to match your breathing rhythm.

✓ Buddy Breathing : Pair up with a friend or family member and practice counting breaths together, taking turns leading the count.

Reflection Questions

✓ How did counting your breaths make you feel?

✓ Did you find it easier to focus and relax?

✓ When might this breathing technique be helpful in your daily life?

Count Your Breath

Activity : Make Your Own Dragon and Practice Dragon Breathing

Objective : To create a fun dragon craft and use it to practice a powerful breathing technique.

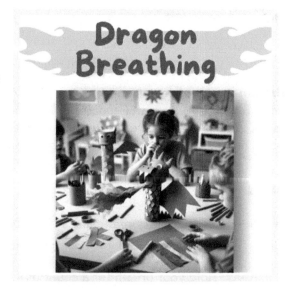

Materials Needed

✓ A toilet paper roll or paper towel roll

✓ Green construction paper

✓ Glue and scissors

✓ Markers or crayons

✓ Red, orange, and yellow tissue paper

✓ Tape

Explanation : Dragon breathing is a powerful breath exercise that can help release tension and stress. By using strong breaths, you can increase the oxygen flow to your brain, which helps improve concentration and energy levels.

Steps

✓ Create Your Dragon :
  • Cover the Roll : Wrap the toilet paper roll with green construction paper and glue it in place.
  • Decorate : Use markers or crayons to draw eyes, scales, and other features on your dragon.

✓ Add Flames :
  • Cut Strips : Cut strips of red, orange, and yellow tissue paper.
  • Attach Flames : Tape the strips to one end of the toilet paper roll to create dragon flames.

- ☑ Dragon Breathing :
  - Position the Dragon : Hold the dragon in front of your mouth.
  - Inhale : Take a deep breath in through your nose.
  - Exhale : Breathe out strongly through your mouth, making the tissue paper flames dance. Imagine you are a powerful dragon breathing out fire!
- ☑ Repeat :
  - Position the Dragon : Practice dragon breathing for a few minutes. Notice how strong breaths help you feel powerful and focused.

Extension Activities

✓ Dragon Stories: Create a story about your dragon. Where does it live? What adventures does it go on?

✓ Breathing Buddies : Pair up with a friend or family member and take turns practicing dragon breathing with each other's dragons.

✓ Dragon Parade : Gather with friends and have a dragon parade, showing off your dragons and practicing dragon breathing together.

Reflection Questions

✓ How did dragon breathing make you feel?

✓ Did you notice any changes in your energy levels or focus?

✓ When might you use dragon breathing in your daily life to help you feel calm and powerful?

Shape Breathing Adventure

Objective : To use shapes to guide your breathing and help you focus on your breath.

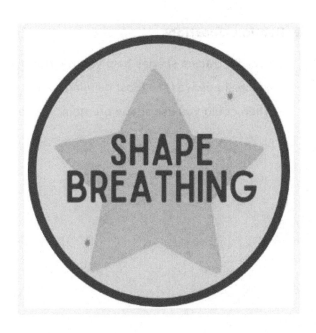

Materials Needed

✓ Paper
✓ Markers or crayons

Explanation : Tracing shapes while breathing helps to create a visual and tactile focus for your breath. This can make it easier to control your breathing rhythm and bring a sense of calm and relaxation.

Steps

- ☑ Draw Shapes :
  - Use the markers or crayons to draw different shapes on a piece of paper, such as a star, heart, square, or circle.

- ☑ Trace and Breathe :
  - Use your finger to trace the outline of a shape.
  - As you trace, breathe in while tracing one side of the shape, and breathe out while tracing the next side.

- ☑ Follow the Pattern :
  - Continue tracing and breathing, following the pattern of the shape.
  - For example, if you are tracing a square, breathe in for one side, out for the next, and repeat.

- ☑ Explore Different Shapes :
  - Try tracing different shapes and notice how it helps you focus on your breath and feel calm.

Extension Activities

- ✓ Create a Shape Book : Draw and color multiple shapes on separate pages and make a booklet to practice shape breathing regularly.

- ✓ Shape Breathing Challenge : Time yourself to see how long you can keep a steady breathing pattern while tracing each shape.

- ✓ Story Shapes : Make up a story for each shape you draw, linking the shapes to different parts of your story to make the activity more engaging.

Reflection Questions

- ✓ How did tracing shapes help you focus on your breathing?
- ✓ Which shape was the most calming for you to trace?
- When could you use shape breathing to help you feel relaxed in your daily life?

Deep Breathing with a Hoberman Sphere

Objective : To explore different breathing techniques for relaxation and stress reduction using a Hoberman sphere.

Materials Needed

✓ Hoberman sphere (expandable ball)

✓ Comfortable seating area

Goals

✓ Learn and practice deep breathing techniques

✓ Increase awareness of breath and body

✓ Promote relaxation and reduce stress

✓ Develop a tool for calming down in stressful situations

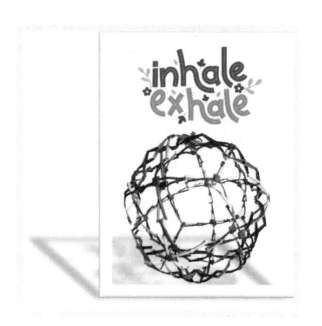

How to Complete

☑ Introduction to Deep Breathing :

- Explain that deep breathing involves taking slow, deep breaths to calm the mind and body. This technique can help reduce stress and promote relaxation

☑ Using the Hoberman Sphere :

- Sit comfortably in a chair or on the floor. Hold the Hoberman sphere in your hands.

- Slowly expand the sphere as you inhale deeply through your nose, filling your lungs with air.

- Hold your breath for a moment, then slowly contract the sphere as you exhale through your mouth, emptying your lungs completely.

☑ Breathing Techniques :

- Box Breathing: Inhale for 4 counts (expand the sphere), hold for 4 counts, exhale for 4 counts (contract the sphere), and hold for 4 counts. Repeat several times.

- 4-7-8 Breathing: Inhale for 4 counts (expand the sphere), hold for 7 counts, exhale for 8 counts (contract the sphere). Repeat several times.

- 5-5-5 Breathing: Inhale for 5 counts (expand the sphere), hold for 5 counts, exhale for 5 counts (contract the sphere). Repeat several times.

- ✔ Practice Deep Breathing :
  - Spend 5-10 minutes practicing deep breathing with the Hoberman sphere. Focus on the movement of the sphere and the rhythm of your breath.
  - Pay attention to how your body feels during and after exercise.

- ✔ Reflect and Discuss :
  - After practicing, reflect on how you feel. Do you feel more relaxed and calm?
  - Discuss your experience with family or friends. Share how deep breathing with the Hoberman sphere helped you relax.

Breath Control Challenge

Objective : To practice controlling breath length and rhythm for relaxation and focus

Materials Needed

✓ Timer or stopwatch

✓ Comfortable seating area

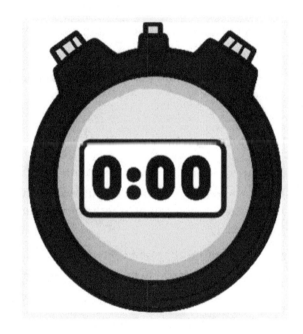

Goals

✓ Improve breath control and awareness

✓ Enhance focus and concentration

✓ Promote relaxation and stress reduction

✓ Develop a tool for calming down in stressful situations

How to Complete

- ✔ Introduction to Breath Control :
  - Explain that controlling your breath length and rhythm can help you stay calm and focused. This activity will challenge you to control your breath in different ways.

Breath Control Exercises :
  - **Long Exhale:** Inhale deeply through your nose for 4 counts, then exhale slowly through your mouth for 8 counts. Repeat several times.

Alternate Nostril Breathing :

- Close your right nostril with your thumb, inhale through your left nostril for 4 counts. Close your left nostril with your finger, release your right nostril, and exhale through your right nostril for 4 counts. Inhale through your right nostril for 4 counts, close it with your thumb, release your left nostril, and exhale through your left nostril for 4 counts. Repeat several times.

Paced Breathing:

- Inhale deeply for 5 counts, hold for 5 counts, exhale for 5 counts, and hold for 5 counts. Repeat several times.

☑ Breath Control Challenge :

- Set a timer for 5-10 minutes. During this time, practice controlling your breath using the exercises above.
- Try to maintain a steady rhythm and focus on your breathing throughout the challenge.

☑ Reflection and Discussion :

- After completing the challenge, reflect on how you felt during the exercises. Did you find it easy or difficult to control your breath?
- Discuss your experience with family or friends. Share which breath control exercise you found most helpful for relaxation and focus.

Additional Breath Control Activities

☑ Balloon Breathing :

- Imagine inflating a balloon as you inhale deeply, filling your lungs completely. Exhale slowly as you imagine the balloon deflating.

☑ Breath of Fire :

- Sit comfortably and take rapid, short breaths through your nose, focusing on quick and forceful exhales. Start slowly and gradually increase the pace.

☑ Humming Breath :

- Inhale deeply and then exhale while humming softly. Notice the vibrations in your chest and throat. Continue for several breaths.

☑ Flower Breathing :

- Imagine smelling a flower as you inhale deeply through your nose, filling your lungs with the scent. Exhale slowly, releasing any tension.

☑ Ocean Breath (Ujjayi) :

- Inhale deeply through your nose, then exhale through your mouth, slightly constricting the back of your throat to create a soft, ocean-like sound. Repeat several times.

- ☑ Rainbow Breathing :
    - Imagine a rainbow in front of you. As you inhale, picture the colors of the rainbow filling your body with calmness. Exhale and release any tension.

- ☑ Breath Counting :
    - Sit comfortably and close your eyes. Inhale and exhale naturally while silently counting each breath. Try to reach a count of 10 without losing focus.

- ☑ Feather Breathing :
    - Hold a feather or imagine holding one. Inhale deeply and then exhale slowly and gently, as if you are trying to keep the feather afloat in the air.

- ☑ Breathing with Music :
    - Play calming music and breathe in sync with the rhythm. Inhale for a certain number of beats and exhale for the same or a different number of beats.

Activity 3: Pulse Oximeter Exploration

Objective : To understand how breathing affects oxygen levels in the body using a pulse oximeter.

Materials Needed

- ✓ Pulse oximeter
- ✓ Comfortable seating area

Goals

- ✓ Learn how breathing impacts oxygen levels in the blood
- ✓ Increase awareness of the connection between breath and body
- ✓ Promote mindfulness and relaxation

How to Complete

- ☑ Introduction to the Pulse Oximeter
    - Explain that a pulse oximeter is a small device that clips onto your finger and measures the oxygen level in your blood and your pulse rate.
    - Show the child how to use the pulse oximeter and explain what the numbers mean.

- ✅ Baseline Measurement
  - Sit comfortably and place the pulse oximeter on your finger. Take a few deep breaths and observe the initial readings for oxygen levels and pulse rate.
  - Write down the baseline measurements.

- ✅ Breathing Exercises
  - Deep Breathing: Practice deep breathing for 5 minutes, then check the pulse oximeter readings. Note any changes in oxygen levels and pulse rate.
  - 4-7-8 Breathing: Perform the 4-7-8 breathing technique for 5 minutes, then check the pulse oximeter readings again. Write down any changes.
  - Alternate Nostril Breathing: Practice alternate nostril breathing for 5 minutes and check the pulseoximeter readings once more.

- ✅ Reflection and Discussion
  - Compare the readings from each breathing exercise to the baseline measurements. Discuss any changes in oxygen levels and pulse rate.
  - Reflect on how different breathing techniques made you feel and how they affected your body.
  - Discuss the importance of mindful breathing for maintaining good oxygen levels and overall health.

Aroma Adventure: Exploring Smells

Objective: To explore different smells and understand how they can affect your mood and calmness.

Materials Needed

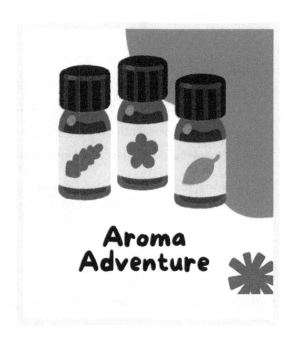

Aroma Adventure

- ✓ Small containers or cotton balls
- ✓ Multiple different scents, such as:

  - Food: vanilla extract, cinnamon, lemon, chocolate, coffee, strawberry, banana, coconut, peanut butter, orange
  - Nature Scents: pine, fresh-cut grass, ocean breeze, rose, lavender, rain, forest, fresh air, wildflowers, autumn leaves
  - Herbs: mint, basil, rosemary, thyme, sage, oregano, parsley, cilantro, dill, chives

Explanation : Our sense of smell is closely linked to our emotions and memories. Remember that smell goes directly to the brain via the olfactory lobe first. This is why certain scents can help us feel more relaxed, focused, or happy. Exploring different smells can enhance your awareness and help you discover which scents help you feel calm.

Steps

✓ Prepare the Scents: Place a few drops of each scent on a cotton ball or in a small container. Label each container with the name of the scent.

✓ Explore the Scents: Have the children sit comfortably and close their eyes. Pass around each scent one at a time, asking them to take a deep breath and describe how the scent makes them feel.

✓ Discuss the Effects: After exploring each scent, discuss how it made them feel. Use questions like:

- "How did you feel when you first smelled the scent?
- Did the scent remind you of any place or time?
- What feelings did you notice when you smelled it?
- Did the scent make you feel calm, happy, or something else?
- How did your body feel when you smelled it? Relaxed or full of energy?
- Was the scent strong or light? How did that make you feel?
- If the scent were a color, what color would it be? Why?
- Did you like the scent? What did you like or not like about it?
- Would you like to smell this scent again? When would you want to smell it?
- How can different smells help you feel better when you're sad or stressed?
- What other things does this scent make you think of?
- Do you think this scent would be good for helping you fall asleep or wake up? Why?
- Can you think of a story that matches this scent?
- What other scents do you know that make you feel happy or calm?
- How would you describe this scent to a friend?

✓ Create a Scent Journal: Provide notebooks or paper for the children to draw or write about their "Aroma Adventure." Encourage them to illustrate their favorite scents and how each one made them feel.

Aroma Adventure: Exploring Smells

Activity: Feather, Whistle, and Object Blowing

Objective : To demonstrate the power of breath through fun activities using feathers, whistles, and other objects.

Materials Needed

✓ Feathers

✓ Whistles

✓ Pinwheels

✓ Straws

✓ Cotton balls

✓ Paper cups

✓ Small light objects (e.g., pom-poms, leaves)

✓ Bubble solution and wands

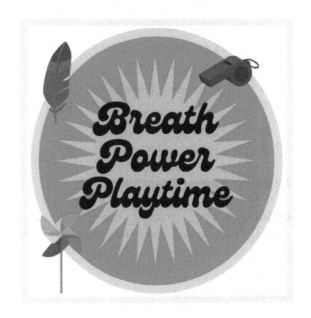

Explanation: Blowing different objects with your breath can help you understand the strength and control of your breath. It also helps you see how breath can be a powerful tool for relaxation and focus.

Steps

✔ Feather Blowing :

- Give each child a feather. Ask them to take a deep breath in and then blow the feather gently, trying to keep it in the air as long as possible.

- Discuss how controlled and gentle breaths can keep the feather floating.

✔ Whistle Blowing :

- Give each child a whistle. Ask them to take a deep breath and blow into the whistle.

- Discuss how strong breaths produce a loud sound, showing the power of their breath.

✔ Pinwheel Spinning :

- Give each child a pinwheel. Ask them to blow on the pinwheel to make it spin.

- Discuss how both gentle and strong breaths can make the pinwheel move at different speeds.

✔ Cotton Ball Race :

- Set up a racetrack with paper cups as obstacles. Give each child a straw and a cotton ball.

- Ask them to use their breath to blow the cotton ball through the racetrack.

- Discuss how controlling their breath can help them navigate the cotton ball around obstacles.

✔ Object Blowing :

- Provide small light objects like pom-poms or leaves. Ask the children to blow the objects across a table or floor.

- Discuss how different objects move differently based on the strength and control of their breath.

- ✔ Bubble Blowing :
  - Give each child a bubble wand and bubble solution. Ask them to take a deep breath and blow gently to create bubbles.
  - Discuss how gentle breaths create bubbles, showing how breath can be soft and controlled.

Flower Breathing Activity

Activity: Flower Breathing

Objective : To practice deep breathing using a creative visualization technique to promote relaxation and mindfulness.

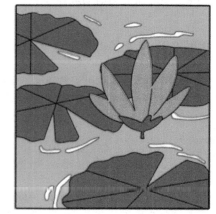

Materials Needed

- ✔ Real or artificial flowers (or pictures of flowers)
- ✔ A quiet, comfortable space
- ✔ Optional: Essential oils with floral scents

Explanation : Flower Breathing is a simple and effective breathing exercise that helps you to slow down, relax, and become more mindful. By visualizing and mimicking the action of smelling a flower, you can focus on your breath and calm your mind

Steps

- ✔ Get Comfortable
  - Find a quiet and comfortable place to sit or stand. If you have real or artificial flowers, hold one in your hand. If not, you can simply imagine your favorite flower.

- ✔ Introduction to Flower Breathing
  - Explain to the children that they will be practicing a breathing exercise called Flower Breathing. They will imagine smelling a beautiful flower to help them focus on their breath and feel calm.

- ✔ Visualize the Flower
  - Ask the children to close their eyes and visualize a beautiful flower. They can choose any flower they like – a rose, a daisy, a tulip, or any other favorite flower.

Inhale Slowly

- Guide the children to take a slow, deep breath in through their nose as if they are smelling the flower. Encourage them to imagine the pleasant scent of the flower filling their lungs.

- Optional : If using essential oils, place a drop on the flower or a cotton ball and let the children smell it as they breathe in.

Hold the Breath

- Ask the children to hold their breath for a moment, savoring the imagined scent of the flower.

Exhale Slowly

- Guide the children to slowly exhale through their mouth, letting go of any tension or stress. Encourage them to imagine blowing the petals of the flower gently.

Repeat Exhale Slowly

- Repeat the process for several breaths, encouraging the children to focus on the calming sensation of the exercise.

Discussion

- After the exercise, discuss how the children felt during Flower Breathing. Use questions like:
  - "How did it feel to imagine smelling the flower?"
  - "Did the exercise help you feel more relaxed?"
  - "What was your favorite part of Flower Breathing?"

Additional Flower Breathing Variations

Flower Breathing with Drawing

- Provide paper and crayons or markers.
- Ask the children to draw their favorite flower before starting the breathing exercise.
- Use their drawings as a visual aid during the exercise.

Flower Breathing with Music

- Play calming, nature-inspired music in the background.
- Let the children listen to music while practicing Flower Breathing, enhancing the relaxation experience.

Flower Breathing with Movement

- Combine Flower Breathing with gentle movements.
- As the children inhale, ask them to raise their arms slowly like a blooming flower.
- As they exhale, ask them to lower their arms gently, imagining the petals closing.

Candle Power Breathing

Objective : To demonstrate the effect of breath and oxygen on a flame and compare it to a battery-powered candle.

Materials Needed

✓ Real candles

✓ Battery-powered candles

✓ Matches or a lighter (for adult use only)

✓ A safe, controlled area for lighting candles

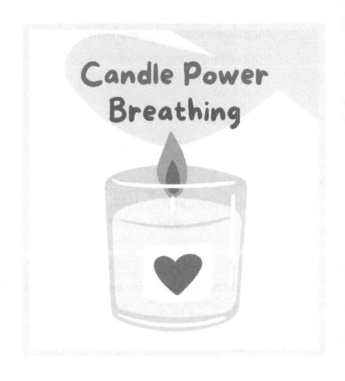

Explanation : Blowing on a candle flame demonstrates how our breath can extinguish a flame by disrupting the supply of oxygen. This activity helps children understand the power of their breath and how it affects the environment around them. Visualizing breath can increase mindfulness of breathing and awareness about how important oxygen is to the brain.

Steps

✓ Safety First
  - Explain the importance of safety when using real candles. Ensure an adult is present to handle lighting and extinguishing the candles.

✓ Lighting the Candle
  - Light a real candle and place it on a stable surface.
  - Place a battery-powered candle next to it for comparison.

✓ Blowing Out the Candle
  - Ask each child to take a deep breath and blow gently on the real candle to extinguish the flame.
  - Discuss how their breath affected the flame and caused it to go out by removing the oxygen it needed to burn.

✓ Comparing with Battery-Powered Candle
  - Ask the children to blow on the battery-powered candle. Point out that it does not go out because it does not need oxygen to stay lit.
  - Discuss the difference between the real candle and the battery-powered candle, emphasizing the role of oxygen and breath.

Discussion

✅ Improved Focus and Concentration

- Discuss how understanding controlled breathing helps to increase oxygen flow to the brain. This can help children realize the importance of deep breathing. Talk about how oxygen improves their ability to focus and improves concentration during schoolwork or other tasks that require attention.

✅ Stress Relief and Emotional Regulation

- Learning to control their breath and seeing a visual effect, like blowing out a candle, can empower children to use breathing techniques to manage stress and regulate their emotions. This skill can help them calm down during stressful situations or when they feel overwhelmed.

Humming Happiness: Vagus Nerve Activation

Activity: Humming Happiness

Objective : To stimulate the vagus nerve through humming and understand how it can help with relaxation and calmness.

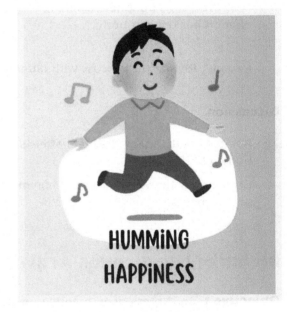

Materials Needed

✓ A quiet, comfortable place to sit

✓ A list of simple songs or tunes to hum

Explanation : The vagus nerve is a key part of our parasympathetic nervous system, which helps us relax and feel calm. It connects the brain to various organs in the body, including the heart, lungs, and digestive tract. Stimulating the vagus nerve through activities like humming can promote relaxation, reduce stress, and enhance overall well-being. The vibrations from humming send signals through the vagus nerve, encouraging the body to enter a state of calm.

Steps

✓ Get Comfortable : Find a quiet and comfortable place to sit.

✓ Choose a Tune : Select a simple song or tune to hum. Examples include :

- "Twinkle, Twinkle, Little Star"
- "Mary Had a Little Lamb"
- "Row, Row, Row Your Boat"
- "Happy Birthday"

- "Baa Baa Black Sheep"
- "Jingle Bells"
- "Old MacDonald Had a Farm"
- "The Alphabet Song"
- "London Bridge is Falling Down"
- "Itsy Bitsy Spider"

✓ **Inhale Deeply** : Take a deep breath in through your nose.

✓ **Hum While Exhaling** : As you exhale, hum the chosen tune, or note. Feel the vibration in your chest and throat

✓ **Feel the Calm** : Continue humming for a few minutes, paying attention to the vibrations and the calming effect it has on your body.

✓ **Repeat** : Repeat the process with different tunes or notes, noticing how each one feels.

Discussion

✓ Ask the children how they feel after humming. Did they notice any changes in their mood or how their body felt?

✓ Explain how the vibrations from humming can stimulate the vagus nerve, helping to promote relaxation and calmness.

Breath of Life Creation Activity

Objective : To express deep breathing experiences creatively through art and reflection.

Materials Needed

✓ Large sheets of paper or canvas

✓ Paints (watercolors, acrylics, or finger paints)

✓ Brushes, sponges, and other painting tools

✓ Crayons, markers, or colored pencils

✓ Glitter, stickers, and other decorative items

✓ Music (optional, for a calming background)

✓ A comfortable space for creating art

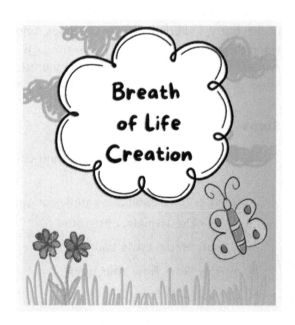

Explanation : This activity encourages children to use art to represent their deep breathing experiences. By translating their feelings and sensations into visual form, they can gain a deeper understanding of how breathing affects their body and mind. This creative process can also be a fun and relaxing way to reflect on the power of their breath.

Steps

☑ Set Up the Space

- Find a comfortable space where children can spread out and create their art. Lay down protective coverings if using paints.
- Play calming music in the background to create a relaxing atmosphere.

☑ Introduction to the Activity

- Explain that they will be using art to express how deep breathing makes them feel. Encourage them to think about the sensations in their body and the emotions they experience while practicing deep breathing.

☑ Deep Breathing Exercise

- Start with a brief deep breathing exercise to help them get in touch with their breath. Guide them through a few minutes of slow, deep breaths, paying attention to how their body feels with each inhale and exhale.

☑ Create Your Breath of Life Art

- Provide each child with a large sheet of paper or canvas and a variety of art supplies.
- Encourage them to use colors, shapes, and textures to represent their breathing experiences. They can paint flowing lines to represent the movement of air, use soothing colors to show relaxation, or create abstract shapes that express their emotions.
- Remind them that there is no right or wrong way to create their art; it is all about personal expression.

☑ Add Decorations

- After they finish their paintings or drawings, provide additional decorative items like glitter, stickers, and other embellishments to enhance their artwork.
- Encourage them to think about how these decorations can add to the story of their breathing experience.

☑ Reflection and Sharing

- Once the art pieces are completed, gather the children in a circle to share their creations.
- Ask each child to describe their artwork and explain how it represents their deep breathing experience. Use questions like:
  - "What colors did you choose and why?"
  - "How does your artwork show the way deep breathing makes you feel?"
  - "What did you learn about your breath through this activity?"

Additional Activities for Reflection

Activity : Breath Journal

Objective : To reflect on deep breathing experiences through writing or drawing in a journal.

Materials Needed

✓ Journals or notebooks

✓ Pens, pencils, crayons, or markers

Explanation : Keeping a journal allows children to regularly reflect on their breathing practices and how it affects their emotions and body. This can help reinforce the benefits of deep breathing and provide a personal space for ongoing exploration.

Steps

☑ Introduction to Journaling
- Explain that they will be starting a Breath Journal to document their deep breathing experiences and reflections.

☑ Journaling Prompts
- Provide prompts to help them get started. Examples include:
    - "Today, when I practiced deep breathing, I felt…"
    - "The colors that remind me of deep breathing are…"
    - "When I breathe deeply, my body feels…"
    - "Something new I noticed about my breath today is…"

☑ Regular Entries
- Encourage them to make regular entries in their journal, whether it is daily, weekly, or after each deep breathing session.

Conclusion : Congratulations! You have learned some amazing techniques to power up your calm throughout this chapter. Remember, you can use these activities anytime you need to relax, focus, or just feel a little bit better. Keep practicing, and you will become a breathing and scent superhero in no time! Your breath and sense of smell are powerful tools that can help you stay calm, relaxed, and ready for anything.

CHAPTER - 7

LISTEN UP

The Magic of Hearing

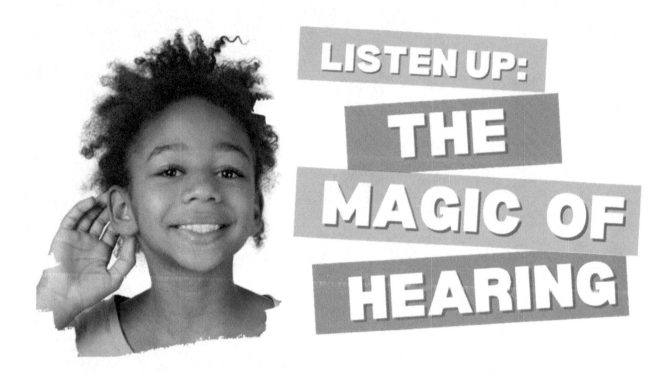

- **Introduction :** Welcome to Chapter 7 of your interoception adventure! In this chapter, we are going to explore the fascinating world of hearing and listening. Hearing is one of our eight senses that helps us detect sounds around us, while listening is an active process where we focus on and interpret these sounds. By practicing listening, we can improve our concentration, calm our minds, and enhance our overall well-being. Get ready to have fun with some exciting listening activities!

The Sound Safari - Outdoor Listening Adventure

Objective : To explore and identify different sounds in nature and become more aware of the environment.

Materials Needed

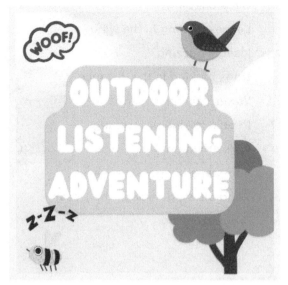

✓ A quiet outdoor space (e.g., park, backyard, nature trail) OR sound clips of outdoor sounds such as birds or weather (rain, wind, thunder)

✓ Notebooks or paper

✓ Pencils or crayons

✓ Small blankets or mats to sit on (optional)

Explanation

Going on an outdoor listening adventure helps children become more aware of their surroundings and appreciate the variety of sounds in nature. This activity encourages mindfulness and enhances their listening skills.

Steps

☑ Find a Quiet Spot

• Take the children to a quiet outdoor space. Ask them to find a comfortable spot to sit and be still.

☑ Listening Session

• Explain that they will be sitting quietly and listening to the sounds around them for a few minutes. Encourage them to close their eyes to focus better on the sounds.

☑ Identify Sounds

• After a few minutes, ask the children to open their eyes and share the sounds they heard. Use questions like :
    • "What sounds did you notice?"
    • "Did you hear any birds or insects?"
    • "What other sounds did you hear, like wind or rustling leaves?"

☑ Draw or Write

• Provide notebooks or paper and ask the children to draw or write about the sounds they heard. They can create a "sound map" of their surroundings.

Examples of Outdoor Sounds

✓ Birds chirping

✓ Leaves rustling in the wind

✓ Insects buzzing

✓ Dogs barking in the distance

✓ Water flowing in a stream

✓ People talking or laughing

✓ Cars driving by

✓ Footsteps on gravel or leaves

✓ Wind blowing through the trees

✓ Frogs croaking

Rhythm Rumble

Activity : Musical Rhythms

Objective : To explore different rhythms, beats in music, and understand how they can affect our mood and energy levels.

Materials Needed

✓ A variety of music with different rhythms (e.g., fast, slow, upbeat, calming)

✓ Speakers or a music player

✓ Space to dance or move around

Explanation

Listening to music with different rhythms helps children understand how sounds can influence their feelings and energy levels. This activity is both fun and educational, promoting an appreciation for music and rhythm.

Steps

✓ Play Different Rhythms
   - Play different types of music with varying rhythms. Start with slow, calming music and then switch to fast, upbeat music.

- ✓ Move to the Music
  - Encourage the children to move or dance to the music. Ask them to notice how their bodies want to move with each rhythm.

- ✓ Discussion
  - After listening to each type of music, discuss how it made them feel. Use questions like :
    - "How did the slow music make you feel?"
    - "Did the fast music make you want to dance?"
    - "Which rhythm was your favorite and why?"

- ✓ Create Your Own Rhythm
  - Provide instruments or household items (like pots, pans, or shakers) and let the children create their own rhythms. Encourage them to experiment with different beats and sounds.

Examples of Music Types and Rhythms

- ✓ Classical Music (Slow and Calming)
  - "Clair de Lune" by Claude Debussy
  - "Moonlight Sonata" by Ludwig van Beethoven
  - "Canon in D" by Johann Pachelbel
  - "Gymnopédie No.1" by Erik Satie
  - "The Swan" by Camille Saint-Saëns

- ✓ Rock Music (Fast and Energetic)
  - "We Will Rock You" by Queen
  - "Eye of the Tiger" by Survivor
  - "Rock and Roll All Nite" by KISS
  - "Born to Be Wild" by Steppenwolf
  - "Livin' on a Prayer" by Bon Jovi

- ✓ Jazz (Varied Rhythms and Beats)
  - "Take Five" by Dave Brubeck
  - "So What" by Miles Davis
  - "Sing, Sing, Sing" by Benny Goodman
  - "A Night in Tunisia" by Dizzy Gillespie
  - "In the Mood" by Glenn Miller

- Pop Music (Upbeat and Catchy)
  - "Happy" by Pharrell Williams
  - "Shake It Off" by Taylor Swift
  - "Uptown Funk" by Mark Ronson ft. Bruno Mars
  - "Can't Stop the Feeling!" by Justin Timberlake
  - "Firework" by Katy Perry

- Hip-hop (Strong Beats and Rhythms)
  - "Can't Hold Us" by Macklemore & Ryan Lewis
  - "Lose Yourself" by Eminem
  - "Sicko Mode" by Travis Scott
  - "HUMBLE." by Kendrick Lamar
  - "Old Town Road" by Lil Nas X

- Reggae (Steady and Relaxing)
  - "Three Little Birds" by Bob Marley
  - "Red, Red Wine" by UB40
  - "One Love" by Bob Marley
  - "I Can See Clearly Now" by Jimmy Cliff
  - "Buffalo Soldier" by Bob Marley

- Country Music (Moderate Tempo)
  - "Jolene" by Dolly Parton
  - "Take Me Home, Country Roads" by John Denver
  - "Ring of Fire" by Johnny Cash
  - "Friends in Low Places" by Garth Brooks
  - "Life is a Highway" by Tom Cochrane

- Electronic Dance Music (Fast and High Energy)
  - "Titanium" by David Guetta ft. Sia
  - "Wake Me Up" by Avicii
  - "Animals" by Martin Garrix
  - "Don't You Worry Child" by Swedish House Mafia
  - "Clarity" by Zedd ft. Foxes

- Folk Music (Steady and Melodic)
  - "The Times They Are A-Changin'" by Bob Dylan
  - "Scarborough Fair" by Simon & Garfunkel
  - "This Land is Your Land" by Woody Guthrie
  - "If I Had a Hammer" by Peter, Paul, and Mary
  - "Blowin' in the Wind" by Bob Dylan

- Lullabies (Slow and Soothing)
  - "Twinkle, Twinkle, Little Star"
  - "Brahms' Lullaby"
  - "Hush, Little Baby"
  - "Rock-a-Bye Baby"
  - "You Are My Sunshine"

Household Harmony

Activity : Sound Makers

Objective : To create different sounds using household items and understand how sounds are produced.

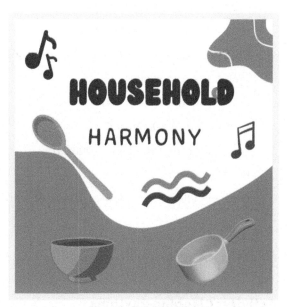

Materials Needed

- Various household items (e.g., pots, pans, spoons, rubber bands, containers, rice, or beans)
- Craft supplies (optional, for decorating instruments)

Explanation

Making sounds with household items helps children learn about sound production and encourages creativity. This activity allows them to explore different types of sounds and understand how they are made.

Steps

- Gather Materials
  - Collect various household items that can be used to make sounds. Examples include pots, pans, spoons, rubber bands, and containers filled with rice or beans.

☑ Create Instruments
  • Let the children experiment with creating different sounds using the items. They can use spoons to tap on pots, shake containers with rice, or stretch rubber bands over boxes to pluck.

☑ Decorate Instruments (Optional)
  • Provide craft supplies for the children to decorate their homemade instruments.

☑ Sound Exploration
  • Encourage the children to play their instruments and explore the different sounds they can make. Ask them to notice the differences in pitch, volume, and tone.

☑ Sound Concert
  • Have the children come together and create a "Household Harmony" concert, where they play their homemade instruments and share the sounds they created.

Examples of Household Items for Sound Makers

✓ Pots and pans (drums)

✓ Wooden spoons (drumsticks)

✓ Rubber bands (guitar strings)

✓ Empty containers with rice or beans (shakers)

✓ Metal lids (cymbals)

✓ Plastic bottles (maracas)

✓ Cardboard tubes (horns)

✓ Aluminum foil (crackling sounds)

✓ Keys (jingles)

✓ Glasses filled with different levels of water (xylophone)

Clap It Out

Activity : Clapping Rhythms

Objective : To explore different rhythms through clapping and understand how rhythm can create patterns in sound.

Materials Needed

✓ Hands (for clapping)

✓ Optional: a metronome or a drum for keeping time

Explanation : Clapping different rhythms helps children understand patterns in music and sound. This activity can improve their sense of timing and rhythm, making them more aware of how different beats affect music and movement.

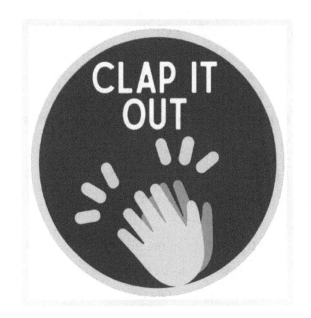

Steps

- Introduce Basic Rhythms
  - Start with simple clapping patterns. For example :
    - Clap-Clap-Pause-Clap-Clap (Clap-Clap-_-Clap-Clap)
    - Clap-Pause-Clap-Clap-Pause-Clap (Clap--Clap-Clap--Clap)

- Follow the Leader
  - Have the children follow your lead as you clap different rhythms. Gradually increase the complexity of the patterns.

- Clap Along to Music
  - Play a song with a clear beat and ask the children to clap along to the rhythm. They can start with slow songs and move to faster ones.

- Create Your Own Rhythms
  - Let the children create their own clapping rhythms and share them with the group. Encourage them to be creative and produce unique patterns.

- Incorporate Other Sounds
  - Add tapping (on a table or the floor) and snapping to the clapping patterns. This can add variety and make the activity more engaging.

Examples of Clapping Patterns

- ✓ Basic : Clap-Clap-Pause-Clap-Clap (Clap-Clap-_-Clap-Clap)
- ✓ Intermediate : Clap-Pause-Clap-Clap-Pause-Clap (Clap--Clap-Clap--Clap)
- ✓ Advanced : Clap-Clap-Snap-Clap-Tap-Clap-Clap-Snap (Clap-Clap-Snap-Clap-Tap-Clap-Clap-Snap)
- ✓ Slow Rhythm : Clap-Pause-Clap-Pause (Clap--Clap-)
- ✓ Fast Rhythm : Clap-Clap-Clap-Clap-Clap-Clap-Clap-Clap (Clap-Clap-Clap-Clap-Clap-Clap-Clap-Clap)
- ✓ Syncopated Rhythm : Clap-Pause-Pause-Clap-Clap-Pause (Clap---Clap-Clap-_)Echo Rhythm: Leader claps a pattern, children echo it back
- ✓ Echo Rhythm : Leader claps a pattern, children echo it back

- ✓ Marching Rhythm : Clap-Clap-Tap-Clap-Clap-Tap (Clap-Clap-Tap-Clap-Clap-Tap)
- ✓ Alternating Claps : Clap-Tap-Clap-Tap (Clap-Tap-Clap-Tap)
- ✓ Double Time : Clap-Clap-Clap-Clap (quickly) (Clap-Clap-Clap-Clap)

Examples of Songs for Clapping Rhythms

- ✓ "We Will Rock You" by Queen
- ✓ "Happy" by Pharrell Williams
- ✓ "If You're Happy and You Know It"
- ✓ "Jingle Bells"
- ✓ "The Wheels on the Bus"
- ✓ "Uptown Funk" by Mark Ronson ft. Bruno Mars
- ✓ "HandClap" by Fitz and The Tantrums
- ✓ "Can't Stop the Feeling!" by Justin Timberlake
- ✓ "Macarena" by Los Del Rio
- ✓ "Shake It Off" by Taylor Swift
- ✓ "Clap Your Hands" by Sia
- ✓ "Footloose" by Kenny Loggins
- ✓ "Shake Your Sillies Out" by The Wiggles
- ✓ "ABC" by The Jackson 5
- ✓ "Don't Stop Believin'" by Journey
- ✓ "We Are Family" by Sister Sledge
- ✓ "Walking on Sunshine" by Katrina and the Waves
- ✓ "Celebration" by Kool & The Gang
- ✓ "Little Bitty Pretty One" by Thirston Harris
- ✓ "I Gotta Feeling" by The Black Eyed Peas

Snapping Fun

Activity : Snapping Rhythms

Objective : To explore different rhythms through snapping fingers and understand how rhythm can create patterns in sound.

Materials Needed

- ✓ Hands (for snapping)
- ✓ Optional: a metronome or a drum for keeping time

Explanation : Snapping different rhythms helps children understand patterns in music and sound. This activity can improve their sense of timing and rhythm, making them more aware of how different beats affect music and movement.

Steps

- ☑ Introduce Basic Snapping
  - Start with simple snapping patterns. For example:
    - Snap-Snap-Pause-Snap-Snap (Snap-Snap-_-Snap-Snap)
    - Snap-Pause-Snap-Snap-Pause-Snap (Snap--Snap-Snap--Snap)

- ☑ Follow the Leader
  - Have the children follow your lead as you snap different rhythms. Gradually increase the complexity of the patterns

- ☑ Snap Along to Music
  - Play a song with a clear beat and ask the children to snap along to the rhythm. They can start with slow songs and move to faster ones.

- ☑ Create Your Own Rhythms
  - Let the children create their own snapping rhythms and share them with the group. Encourage them to be creative and produce unique patterns.

- ☑ Combine with Clapping
  - Combine snapping with clapping patterns to create more complex rhythms.

Examples of Songs for Snapping Rhythms

- ✓ "Under the Sea" from The Little Mermaid
- ✓ "Do-Re-Mi" from The Sound of Music
- ✓ "Sugar, Sugar" by the Archies
- ✓ "You've Got a Friend in Me" from Toy Story
- ✓ "Zip-a-Dee-Doodah"
- ✓ "Happy" by Pharrell Williams
- ✓ "ABC" by The Jackson 5
- ✓ "Witch Doctor" by David Seville
- ✓ "Hakuna Matata" from The Lion King

- ✓ "The Bare Necessities" from The Jungle Book
- ✓ "Supercalifragilisticexpialidocious" from Mary Poppins
- ✓ "Friend Like Me" from Aladdin
- ✓ "Name Game" by Shirley Ellis
- ✓ "Under the Boardwalk" by The Drifters
- ✓ "Stand By Me" by Ben E. King
- ✓ "My Girl" by The Temptations
- ✓ "Lollipop" from Chordettes

Stomping Beats

Activity : Stomping Rhythms

Objective : To explore different rhythms through stomping feet and understand how rhythm can create patterns in sound.

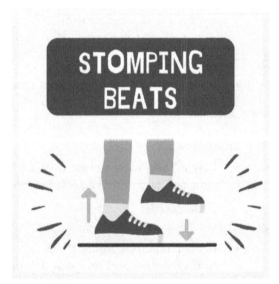

Materials Needed

- ✓ Feet (for stomping)
- ✓ Optional: a metronome or a drum for keeping time

Explanation

Stomping different rhythms helps children understand patterns in music and sound. This activity can improve their sense of timing and rhythm, making them more aware of how different beats affect music and movement.

Steps

- ✓ Introduce Basic Stomping
  - Start with simple stomping patterns. For example :
    - Stomp-Stomp-Pause-Stomp-Stomp (Stomp-Stomp-_-Stomp-Stomp)
    - Stomp-Pause-Stomp-Stomp-Pause-Stomp (Stomp--Stomp-Stomp--Stomp)

- ✓ Follow the Leader
  - Have the children follow your lead as you stomp different rhythms. Gradually increase the complexity of the patterns.

- ☑ Stomp Along to Music
  - Play a song with a clear beat and ask the children to stomp along to the rhythm. They can start with slow songs and move to faster ones.of the patterns.

- ☑ Create Your Own Rhythms
  - Let the children create their own stomping rhythms and share them with the group. Encourage them to be creative and produce unique patterns.

- ☑ Combine with Clapping and Snapping
  - Combine stomping with clapping and snapping patterns to create more complex rhythms.

Examples of Stomping Patterns

- ✓ Basic : Stomp-Stomp-Pause-Stomp-Stomp (Stomp-Stomp-_-Stomp-Stomp)
- ✓ Intermediate : Stomp-Pause-Stomp-Stomp-Pause-Stomp (Stomp--Stomp-Stomp--Stomp)
- ✓ Advanced : Stomp-Stomp-Clap-Stomp-Tap-Stomp-Stomp-Clap (Stomp-Stomp-Clap-Stomp-Tap-Stomp-Stomp-Clap)
- ✓ Slow Rhythm : Stomp-Pause-Stomp-Pause (Stomp--Stomp-)
- ✓ Fast Rhythm : Stomp-Stomp-Stomp-Stomp-Stomp-Stomp-Stomp-Stomp (Stomp-Stomp-Stomp-Stomp-Stomp-Stomp-Stomp-Stomp)
- ✓ Syncopated Rhythm : Stomp-Pause-Pause-Stomp-Stomp-Pause (Stomp---Stomp-Stomp-_)
- ✓ Echo Rhythm : Leader stomps a pattern, children echo it back
- ✓ Marching Rhythm : Stomp-Stomp-Clap-Stomp-Stomp-Clap (Stomp-Stomp-Clap-Stomp-Stomp-Clap)
- ✓ Alternating Stomps : Stomp-Clap-Stomp-Clap (Stomp-Clap-Stomp-Clap)
- ✓ Double Time : Stomp-Stomp-Stomp-Stomp (quickly) (Stomp-Stomp-Stomp-Stomp)

Examples of Songs for Stomping Rhythms

- ✓ "Waka Waka" by Shakira
- ✓ "I Like to Move It" from Madagascar
- ✓ "We Will Rock You" by Queen
- ✓ "Stomp" by The Brothers Johnson
- ✓ "Shake It Off" by Taylor Swift
- ✓ "Can't Stop the Feeling!" by Justin Timberlake
- ✓ "Happy" by Pharrell Williams
- ✓ "Footloose" by Kenny Loggins
- ✓ "Jump In The Line" by Harry Belafonte
- ✓ "Uptown Funk" by Mark Ronson ft. Bruno Mars
- ✓ "Dynamite" by Taio Cruz

✓ "Eye of the Tiger" by Survivor

✓ "Roar" by Katy Perry

✓ "Get Up Offa That Thing" by James Brown

✓ "Thunder" by Imagine Dragons

✓ "Dance Monkey" by Tones and I

Sound Exploration

Activity : Loud vs. Quiet Sounds

Objective : To explore the differences between loud and quiet sounds and understand how they affect our body and emotions.

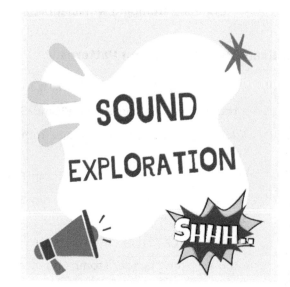

Materials Needed

✓ Various objects or instruments to create loud and quiet sounds (e.g., drum, maracas, bells, shakers)

✓ Space to move around

Explanation

Exploring loud and quiet sounds helps children understand how different volumes can affect their feelings and body sensations. This activity encourages mindfulness and awareness of how sound impacts their emotions and physical state.

Steps

☑ Introduce Loud and Quiet Sounds
  • Demonstrate loud and quiet sounds using different objects or instruments. For example, bang a drum for a loud sound and gently shake a maraca for a quiet sound.

☑ Feel the Sounds
  • Ask the children to close their eyes and feel how their body reacts to loud and quiet sounds. Discuss how the different volumes make them feel.

☑ Move to the Sounds
  • Play loud and quiet sounds and encourage the children to move around. Ask them to move energetically to loud sounds and gently to quiet sounds.

- Create Your Own Sounds
  - Let the children create their own loud and quiet sounds using objects or instruments. Encourage them to experiment with different volumes.

- Discussion
  - After the activity, discuss how the different sounds made them feel. Use questions like:
    - "How did the loud sounds make you feel?"
    - "Did the quiet sounds help you feel calm?"
    - "Which did you prefer, loud or quiet sounds?"

Examples of Loud and Quiet Sounds

- Loud Sounds
- ✓ Banging a drum
- ✓ Clapping hands loudly
- ✓ Shaking a tambourine
- ✓ Blowing a whistle
- ✓ Stomping feet
- ✓ Ringing a loud bell
- ✓ Playing a trumpet
- ✓ Hitting a cymbal
- ✓ Using a loud rattle
- ✓ Yelling

- Quiet Sounds
- ✓ Gently shaking a maraca
- ✓ Softly tapping a triangle
- ✓ Whispering
- ✓ Lightly tapping a drum
- ✓ Rubbing sandpaper blocks together
- ✓ Ringing a small bell
- ✓ Playing a flute softly
- ✓ Tapping a wooden block lightly
- ✓ Using a soft rattle
- ✓ Humming quietly

Conclusion : Congratulations! In this chapter, you have explored the magic of hearing and listening through fun and engaging activities. You have gone on an outdoor listening adventure, experimented with musical rhythms, created your own sounds with household items, explored clapping, snapping, and stomping rhythms, and discovered the effects of loud and quiet sounds. By practicing listening, you have improved your concentration, mindfulness, and appreciation for the sounds around you. Keep exploring the world of sound and remember that listening is a powerful tool that can help you stay connected, calm, and focused.

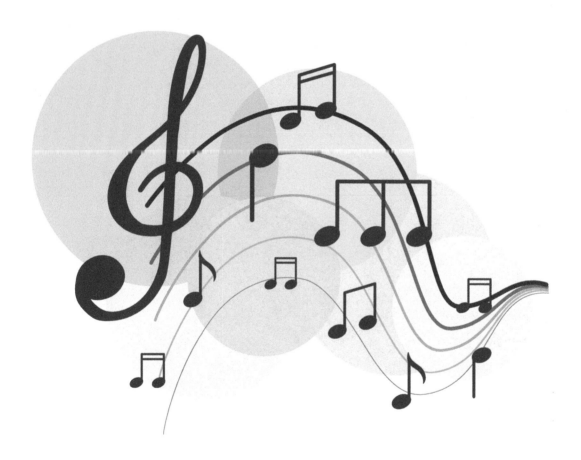

CHAPTER - 8

DReamLaNd aDVeNTUReS

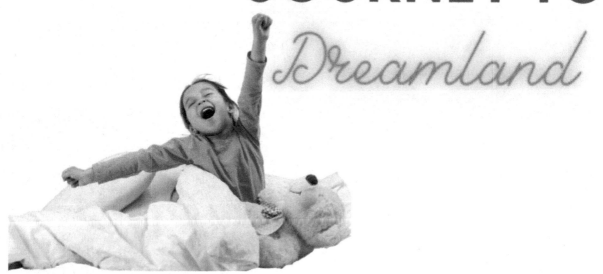

JOURNEY TO
Dreamland

Introduction : Welcome to Chapter 8 of your interoception adventure! In this chapter, we will explore the wonderful world of sleep and its importance for your body and mind. Sleep helps you rest, recharge, and get ready for new adventures. We will learn about the benefits of sleep, the stages of sleep, and fun activities to help you sleep better and feel great!

Why Sleep is Important

Growth and Development : Sleep helps your body grow and develop. While you sleep, your body releases growth hormones that help you become strong and healthy.

Brain Function : Sleep helps your brain work better. It helps you remember things, solve problems, and regulate your emotions. A good night's sleep makes it easier to learn new things.

Emotional Health : Getting enough sleep helps you feel happier and less stressed. It makes it easier to manage daily challenges and enjoy life.

Physical Health : Sleep helps your body fight off illnesses and stay healthy. It also helps maintain a healthy weight and reduces the risk of getting sick.

The Science of Sleep

Sleep Stages : Sleep is divided into several stages, including light sleep (stages 1 and 2), deep sleep (stages 3 and 4), and REM (rapid eye movement) sleep. Each stage plays an important role in making you feel rested and refreshed.

- Light Sleep : The transition from being awake to sleeping. Your body starts to relax and get ready for deeper sleep.

- Deep Sleep : This is when your body does most of its repair and growth. It is essential for feeling rested in the morning.

- REM Sleep : This stage is when you have vivid dreams. It is important for memory, learning, and processing emotions.

Improving Sleep Quality

To help you get the best sleep, it is important to have good sleep habits and a bedtime routine. Here are some tips and fun activities to help you sleep better:

Tranquil Sleep Practices

1. Dreamy Journal

Description : Keep a sleep journal to write or draw about your dreams and how you feel after waking up.

Goal : Reflect on sleep patterns and understand the connection between sleep quality and your daily feelings.

Thrilling Twist : Decorate your journal with stickers and drawings to make it fun and personal.

How to Complete

- ☑ Choose a Journal : Pick a notebook or journal that you like. Decorate the cover with stickers, drawings, or photos to make it special.

- ☑ Daily Entries : Each morning, write or draw about your dreams from the night before. Include details like colors, people, and places you remember.

- ☑ Feelings Check : Write down how you feel when you wake up. Are you tired, happy, or grumpy?

- ☑ Patterns: After a week, look for patterns. Do you notice that you feel better after nights with certain types of dreams?

- ☑ Share: Share your favorite dream entries with family or friends.

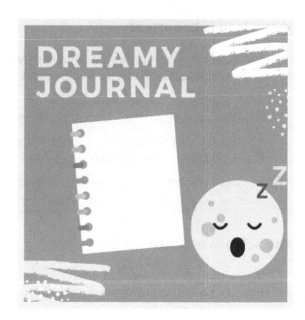

Bedtime Routine Race

Description : Turn your bedtime routine into a fun race. Create a checklist of activities like brushing your teeth, reading a book, and putting on pajamas. See how quickly you can complete each task while still relaxing.

Goal : Establish a consistent bedtime routine to signal to your body that it is time to sleep.

Thrilling Twist : Offer small rewards for completing the routine consistently over a week, like choosing the next bedtime story or an extra 10 minutes of reading time.

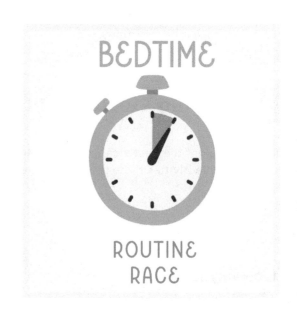

How to Complete

- ☑ Create a Checklist : List your bedtime tasks on a chart (e.g., brushing teeth, washing face, changing into pajamas, reading a book, turning off lights).

- ☑ Set a Timer : Use a timer to see how quickly you can complete each task. Make sure to do each task properly.

- ☑ Race with Family : Turn it into a family activity by racing to see who can finish their bedtime routine the quickest.

- ✓ Track Progress : Keep a chart to track your routine completion times each night.
- ✓ Rewards : Set up a reward system for completing the routine on time for a week, like choosing the next bedtime story or a special treat.

Sleepy Signals

Description : Draw or list the signals that tell you when you are tired (e.g., yawning, rubbing eyes, feeling cranky).

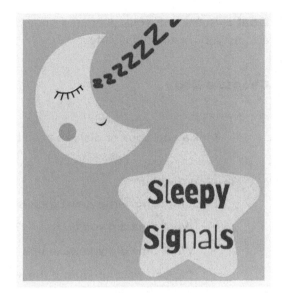

Goal : Learn to recognize the body's signals that it is time to sleep.

Thrilling Twist : Create a "Sleepy Signals" poster to hang in your room.

Make a List : Think about how your body feels when you are tired. Do you yawn, rub your eyes, or feel cranky?

- ✓ Here are some possible signals :

  - Heavy Eyelids : Feeling like your eyelids are drooping.
  - Difficulty Focusing : Finding it hard to concentrate on tasks.
  - Irritability : Becoming easily annoyed or frustrated.
  - Decreased Energy : Feeling low on energy or sluggish.
  - Frequent Blinking : Blinking more often than usual.
  - Fidgeting : Moving around restlessly.
  - Loss of Interest : Losing interest in activities you usually enjoy.
  - Clumsiness : Becoming more prone to dropping things or stumbling.
  - Headaches : Experiencing mild headaches.
  - Mood Swings : Experiencing sudden changes in mood

Create a Poster : Use your drawings or list to create a colorful poster.

Hang It Up : Hang the poster in your room as a reminder to recognize your sleepy signals.

Discuss : Talk with a parent or caregiver about your sleepy signals and what to do when you notice them.

Slumber Log

Description : Keep a log of your slumber by your bed and write down details about your sleep each morning. Note how you felt before going to bed and when you woke up.

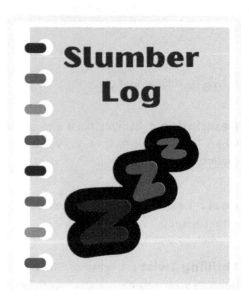

Goal : Reflect on your sleep and understand how it affects your rest and daily life.

Choose a Diary

☑ Introduce Loud and Quiet Sounds
  - Pick a notebook or diary to keep by your bed.

☑ Morning Routine
  - Each morning, write down details about your sleep :
    - What time did you go to bed?
    - What time did you wake up?
    - Did you wake up during the night?
    - How did you feel before going to bed?
    - How did you feel when you woke up?

☑ Reflect
  - Think about your sleep quality.
  - Reflect on how your sleep made you feel.
  - Consider how a good or bad night's sleep might affect your mood for the day.

☑ Extra Reflection Questions
  - Did you have any trouble falling asleep? If so, why do you think that happened?
  - Did you wake up feeling refreshed or still tired?
  - Did you have any thoughts or worries before bed that affected your sleep?
  - What was the most relaxing part of your bedtime routine?
  - Did you notice any difference in your sleep if you did something different before bed, like reading or avoiding screens?
  - How many hours of sleep did you get? Was it more or less than usual?
  - Did you have any physical sensations during sleep, like feeling too hot or cold?
  - Did you hear any noises during the night that disturbed your sleep?
  - Did you have any bedtime snacks or drinks? Did they affect your sleep?
  - How did your sleep affect your energy levels and mood throughout the day?

⊘ Share

- Share your sleep diary with family or friends.

- Create a "Slumber Log" with your observations and reflections.

- Discuss your sleep patterns and how they might improve.

By keeping a sleep log and answering these reflection questions, you'll learn more about your sleep patterns, helping you to get better rest and enjoy more energetic days!

Relaxation Routine

Description : Create a relaxation routine to help you wind down before bed. This could include activities like reading a book, taking a warm bath, or practicing deep breathing. Draw or write about your relaxation routine.

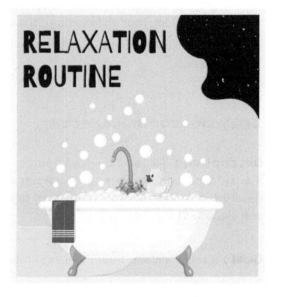

Goal : Promote relaxation before bedtime.

Thrilling Twist : Make a "Relaxation Routine" poster with pictures of your favorite calming activities.

How to Complete

⊘ Choose Activities : List your bedtime tasks on a chart (e.g., brushing teeth, washing face, changing into pajamas, reading a book, turning off lights).

⊘ Create a Schedule : Create a schedule for your relaxation routine, setting aside time for each activity.

⊘ Draw or Write : Draw pictures or write about your relaxation routine.

⊘ Practice Nightly : Practice your relaxation routine each night before bed.

⊘ Reflect : Reflect on how your relaxation routine makes you feel and how it helps you sleep better.

Ideas for Relaxating Activities

✓ Story Time : Read a calming story together.

✓ Nature Walk : Take a walk outside and focus on the sights and sounds of nature.

✓ Bubble Blowing : Blow bubbles and watch them float away, focusing on slow and steady breaths.

✓ Listening to Nature Sounds : Play recordings of nature sounds like rain, birds, or waves.

✓ Yoga : Practice simple yoga poses designed for children.

✓ Guided Imagery : Guide kids through imagining a peaceful and happy place.

✓ **Crafting** : Engage in simple, calming crafts like making friendship bracelets or drawing.

✓ **Soft Toy Cuddle** : Cuddle with a favorite soft toy or blanket.

✓ **Breathing Exercises** : Practice simple breathing exercises, like pretending to blow up a balloon slowly.

✓ **Quiet Time Tent** : Create a small, cozy tent or fort where kids can sit quietly with some soft toys and books.

✓ **Scented Playdough** : Use playdough infused with calming scents like lavender or chamomile.

✓ **Aromatherapy with Essential Oils** : Allow kids to smell different essential oils and pick their favorite calming scent. Make a spray with some water and a few drops of essential oils for bedding.

✓ **Herbal Tea Tasting** : Have a small tea party with caffeine-free herbal teas, letting them taste different flavors like chamomile or peppermint.

✓ **Scent Exploration** : Provide a variety of natural items with different scents (e.g., flowers, herbs, citrus peels) and let your child explore the smells.

✓ **Calming Snacks** : Offer healthy, soothing snacks like warm oatmeal with a hint of cinnamon or a cup of warm milk.

Cozy Bedroom Makeover

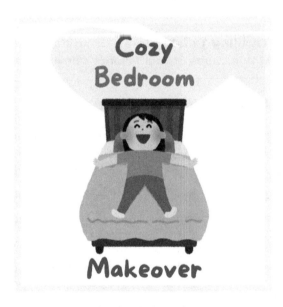

Description : Redecorate your bedroom to make it a cozy and comfortable sleep environment. Draw or describe the changes you made and how they help you sleep better.

Goal : Create a sleep-friendly environment.

Thrilling Twist : Have a "Bedroom Makeover Day" where you get to rearrange and decorate your room.

How to Complete

☑ Assess Your Room : Look around your room and think about what changes could make it cozier and more comfortable.

- Fairy Lights : Hang fairy lights around the room to create a warm, inviting glow.

- Soft Bedding : Choose soft, comfortable bedding in fun colors or patterns that the child loves.

- Stuffed Animals : Add a collection of favorite stuffed animals to the bed or shelves for comfort and decoration.

- Canopy or Tent : Install a bed canopy or play tent to create a cozy nook for reading and relaxing.

- Wall Art : Decorate the walls with colorful artwork, posters of favorite characters, or framed pictures.

- Glow-in-the-Dark Stickers : Use glow-in-the-dark stars and moon stickers on the ceiling to create a magical night sky.

- Rug : Add a soft, plush rug to the floor for extra comfort and a cozy feel.

- Reading Corner : Create a reading corner with a comfortable chair or bean bag, a small bookshelf, and good lighting.

- Pillows : Add plenty of soft pillows in different shapes, sizes, and colors to the bed or reading nook.

- Curtains : Choose blackout curtains to help keep the room dark and improve sleep quality.

- Dream Catcher : Hang a dream catcher above the bed for a whimsical touch and to help with sweet dreams.

- Nightlight : Use a soft, dim nightlight to provide a comforting glow for those who prefer not to sleep in complete darkness.

- Personalized Name Decor : Add personalized decor items like a name sign or initial letters to make the room feel special.

- Storage Solutions : Use colorful bins or baskets to keep toys, books, and clothes organized and tidy.

- Calming Colors : Paint the walls in calming, soothing colors like pastel blues, greens, or lavender.

- Themed Decor : Choose a theme the child loves, like animals, space, or a favorite TV show, and incorporate themed decor items.

- Sensory Items : Add sensory items like a soft blanket, textured pillows, or a weighted blanket for extra comfort.

- DIY Art Projects : Display DIY art projects created by the child to make the room feel more personal and creative.

- Interactive Wall : Create an interactive wall with a chalkboard or whiteboard for drawing and writing.

- Aromatherapy : Use a diffuser with calming essential oils like lavender or chamomile to create a relaxing atmosphere.

☑ Make Changes : Make changes to your room, such as rearranging furniture, adding soft blankets, or putting up calming decorations.

☑ Draw or Describe : Draw pictures or write about the changes you made and how they help you sleep better.

☑ Reflect : Reflect on how your new bedroom setup makes you feel.

☑ Enjoy : Enjoy your new cozy bedroom and notice how it helps improve your sleep.

Nighttime Storytelling

Description : Tell or listen to a bedtime story with your family or friends. Draw or write about the story you heard and how it made you feel.

Goal : Create a peaceful transition to sleep.

Thrilling Twist : Write and illustrate your own bedtime story to share with others.

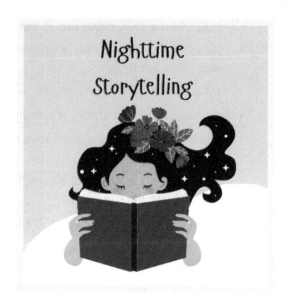

How to Complete

- ⬤ Choose a Story : Choose a bedtime story to read or listen to.

- ⬤ Read Aloud : Read the story aloud with family or friends.

- ⬤ Discuss : Discuss the story and how it made you feel.

- ⬤ Draw or Write : Draw pictures or write about the story you heard.

- ⬤ Create Your Own : Write and illustrate your own bedtime story to share with others.

Here are 15 Suggestions for Bedtime Stories

- ✓ "Goodnight Moon" by Margaret Wise Brown - A classic bedtime story that helps children say goodnight to everything around them.

- ✓ "The Very Quiet Cricket" by Eric Carle - A gentle story about a cricket finding his voice, with beautiful illustrations.

- ✓ "Guess How Much I Love You" by Sam McBratney - A heartwarming tale of the love between Little Nutbrown Hare and Big Nutbrown Hare.

- ✓ "The Tale of Peter Rabbit" by Beatrix Potter - A soothing story of Peter Rabbit's adventures in Mr. McGregor's garden.

- ✓ "Owl Moon" by Jane Yolen - A peaceful story of a father and daughter searching for an owl on a winter night.

- ✓ "The Snowy Day" by Ezra Jack Keats - A calming story about a boy exploring his neighborhood after the first snowfall.

- ✓ "Good Night, Gorilla" by Peggy Rathmann - A delightful and quiet story about a mischievous gorilla and a zookeeper.

- ✓ "Where the Wild Things Are" by Maurice Sendak - Though slightly adventurous, the calming conclusion helps children wind down.

- ✓ "I Love You to the Moon and Back" by Amelia Hepworth - A sweet story about the love between a parent and child.

- ✓ "Llama Llama Red Pajama" by Anna Dewdney - A comforting story about a little llama waiting for his mama at bedtime.

- ✓ "Room on the Broom" by Julia Donaldson - A gentle rhyming story about a kind witch and her animal friends.

- ✓ "The Runaway Bunny" by Margaret Wise Brown - A sweet tale of a mother bunny's unwavering love for her little one.

- ✓ "Brown Bear, Brown Bear, What Do You See?" by Bill Martin Jr. and Eric Carle - A rhythmic and repetitive story that helps children wind down.

- ✓ "The Kissing Hand" by Audrey Penn - A reassuring story about a raccoon named Chester who feels comforted by his mother's kiss.

- ✓ "The Velveteen Rabbit" by Margery Williams - A classic story about a stuffed rabbit's journey to becoming real through the love of a child.

Nighttime Sleepy Scavenger Hunt

Description : Create a scavenger hunt in your bedroom to find items that help you sleep better (e.g., stuffed animals, a cozy blanket, a favorite book). Draw or list the items you found and how they help you relax.

Goal : Identify items that contribute to a good night's sleep.

Thrilling Twist : Make a "Sleepy Scavenger Hunt" map and decorate it with drawings of your favorite sleep items.

How to Complete

- ✓ List Items : Make a list of items in your room that help you sleep better.

- ✓ Create Clues : Create clues for a scavenger hunt to find these items.

- ✓ Search : Follow the clues to find each item in your room.

- ✓ Draw or List : Draw pictures or make a list of the items you found and how they help you relax.

- ✓ Create a Map : Create a scavenger hunt map and decorate it with drawings of your favorite sleep items.

Cozy Comfort Creations: Exploring Weighted Blankets and Stuffed Animals

*Caution: Avoid use of weighted blankets for children who are younger than 2 and for kids who are unable to remove them on their own.

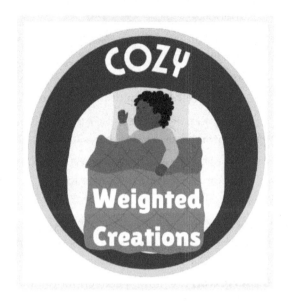

Description : To explore how weighted blankets and stuffed animals can enhance sleep and relaxation, and to understand the benefits of these comforting items.

Materials Needed

- ✓ Weighted blanket
- ✓ Various stuffed animals
- ✓ Comfortable space to lie down
- ✓ Notebooks and crayons or markers

Explanation : Weighted blankets and stuffed animals can provide a sense of security and comfort that helps improve sleep quality. This activity will help you discover how those items make you feel and how they can enhance your bedtime routine.

More About Weighted Items

What Are Weighted Blankets?

- ✓ Weighted blankets are blankets filled with materials like glass beads or plastic pellets to add extra weight. They are designed to be heavier than regular blankets, typically ranging from 5 to 30 pounds.

Benefits of Weighted Blankets

- ✅ Deep Pressure Stimulation (DPS) : The added weight provides gentle, even pressure across the body, like a hug. This can help calm the nervous system and reduce feelings of anxiety.

- ✅ Increased Serotonin and Melatonin : The pressure from weighted blankets can stimulate the production of serotonin, a hormone that promotes relaxation, and melatonin, a hormone that helps regulate sleep.

- ✅ Reduced Anxiety : Many people find that weighted blankets help reduce anxiety and create a feeling of security.

- ✅ Improved Sleep Quality : Weighted blankets can help people fall asleep faster and stay asleep longer, leading to better overall sleep quality.

- ✅ Enhanced Focus and Attention : Some studies suggest that using weighted blankets can improve focus and attention, particularly for individuals with ADHD or sensory processing disorders.

Using Weighted Stuffed Animals

✓ Weighted stuffed animals work on the same principle as weighted blankets, providing a comforting weight that can help soothe and calm.

✓ They are particularly useful for children who may find the full weight of a blanket overwhelming or for those who need a portable source of comfort.

Steps

☑ Introduction to Cozy Comfort Creations

- Explain that you will be exploring how weighted blankets and stuffed animals can help you feel more comfortable and relaxed at bedtime. Share the benefits of using these items, such as reducing anxiety, providing a sense of security, and improving sleep quality.

☑ Try Out the Weighted Blanket

- Find a comfortable place to lie down. Place the weighted blanket over your body and relax for a few minutes. Notice how the blanket feels and how it makes your body feel.

- Optional: Use a regular blanket first and then switch to the weighted blanket to compare the sensations.

☑ Experiment with Stuffed Animals

- Gather a variety of stuffed animals. Choose your favorites and cuddle with them while lying under the weighted blanket or a regular blanket.

- Notice how the stuffed animals make you feel. Do they provide extra comfort or security?

☑ Discussion

- After relaxing with the weighted blanket and stuffed animals, discuss how you felt during the activity. Use questions like :

    - "How did the weighted blanket feel on your body?"

    - "Did you feel more relaxed and secure with the weighted blanket?"

    - "Which stuffed animals made you feel the most comfortable?"

    - "How did using the stuffed animals and weighted blanket together make you feel?"

    - "Would you like to use these items as part of your bedtime routine?"

☑ Create a Cozy Comfort Chart

- Use notebooks and crayons or markers to create a chart. Draw or write about how each item (weighted blanket, different stuffed animals) made you feel.

- Include a rating system (e.g., stars or smiley faces) to rate the comfort and relaxation level of each item.

☑ Share Your Findings

- Share your Cozy Comfort Chart with family or friends. Discuss which items you liked the most and why.

- Consider incorporating your favorite comforting items into your nightly bedtime routine.

Thrilling Twist

☑ Comfort Creature Companions

- Create a bedtime ritual where you choose your favorite stuffed animal and tuck it in with you every night. Name your stuffed animals and tell a bedtime story involving your Comfort Creature Companions.By exploring the cozy comfort of weighted blankets and stuffed animals, you can find new ways to enhance your sleep and create a more relaxing bedtime environment. Enjoy the soothing benefits of these comforting items and sleep well!

Conclusion : By understanding the importance of sleep and incorporating these thrilling activities, you can develop healthy sleep habits that support your overall well-being, growth, and development. With good sleep hygiene and a consistent bedtime routine, you will be ready to energize and recharge, facing each new day with enthusiasm and joy. Sweet dreams!

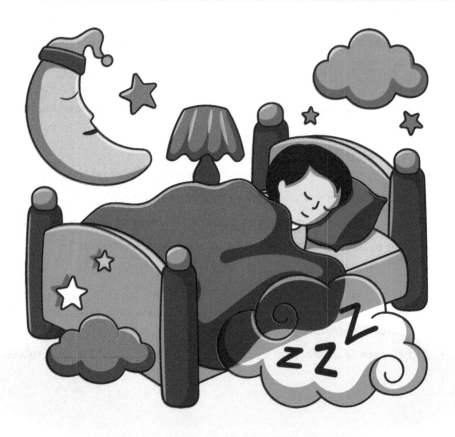

CHaPTeR - 9

ReSOURCeS

- The following chapter contains resources for use in multiple activities throughout this book. Feel free to copy them and use them as long as the original document is not altered in any way.

- Additional activities **and a journal** will be available for purchase and download in the future at CaraKoscinski.com

SCaN The CODe TO DOWNLOaD The ReSOURceS FOR FRee.

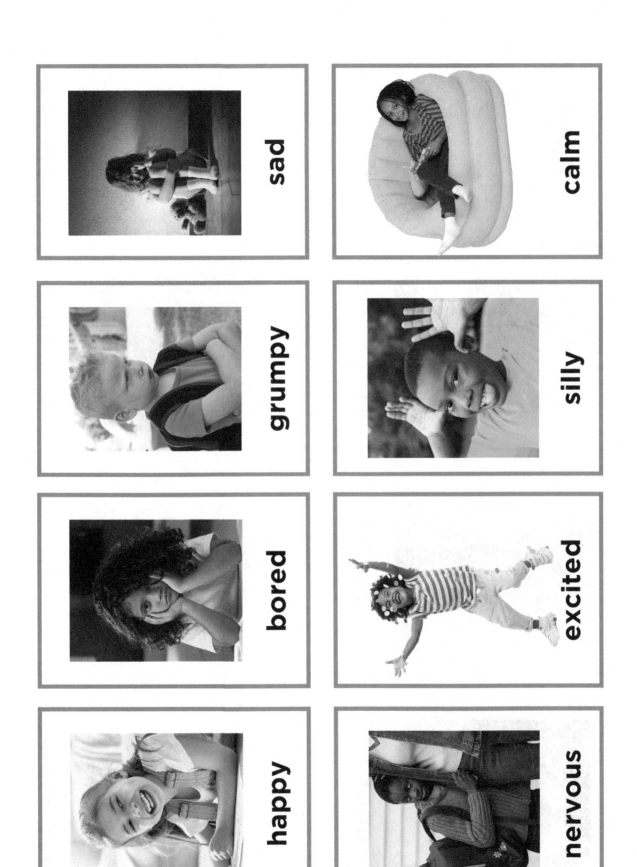

sad

calm

grumpy

silly

bored

excited

happy

nervous

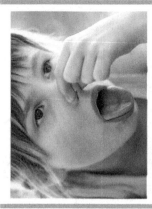 disgusted

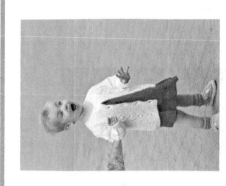 shocked

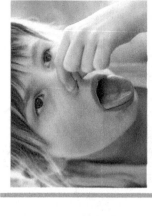 surprised

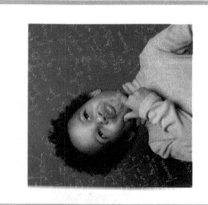 confused

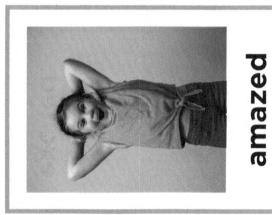 amazed

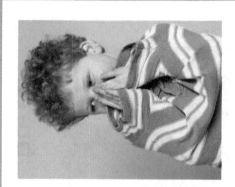 shy

angry

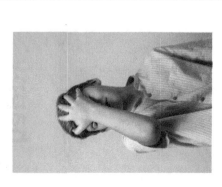 disappointed

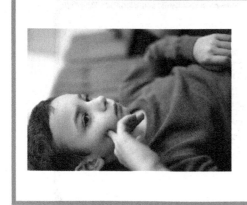

pensive

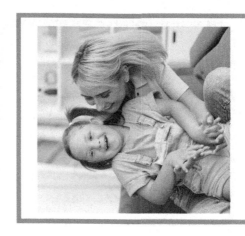

love

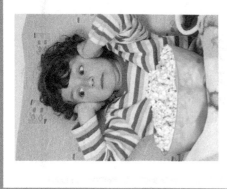

scared

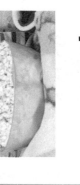

excited

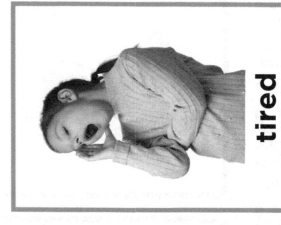

cranky

tired

proud

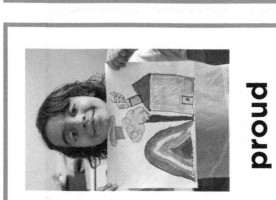

worried

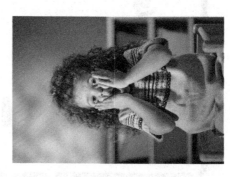

Emotions Cards

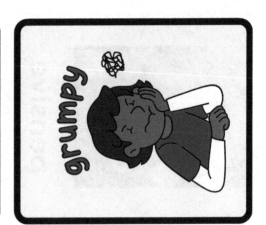

funny

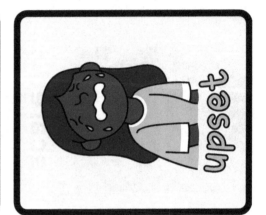

grumpy

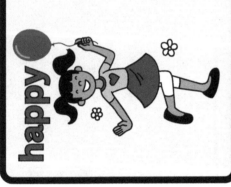

happy

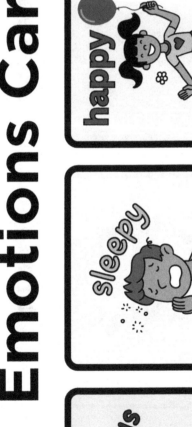

upset

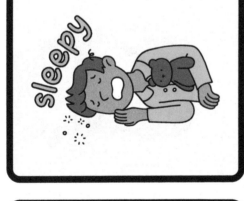

sleepy

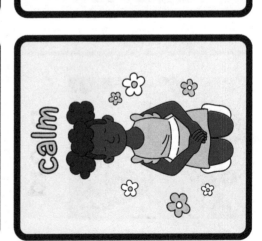

tired

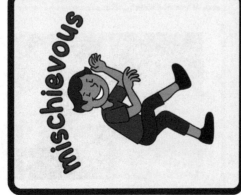

mischievous

calm

Emotions Cards

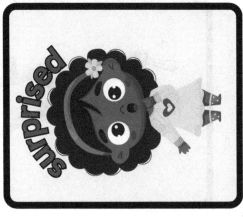

surprised

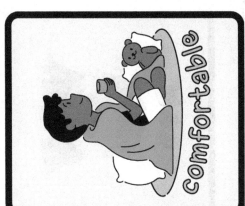

comfortable

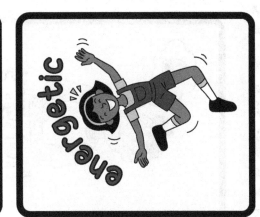

energetic

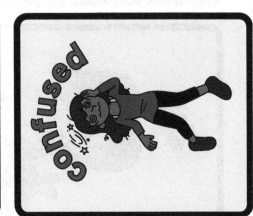

confused

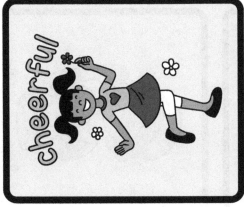

ashamed

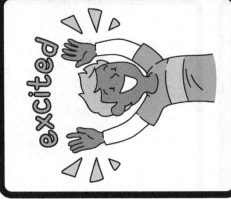

jealous

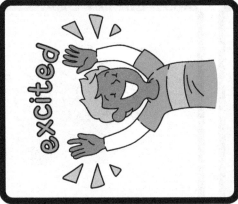

excited

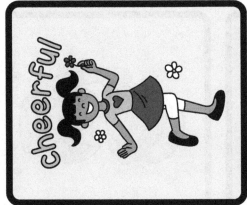

cheerful

Emotions Cards

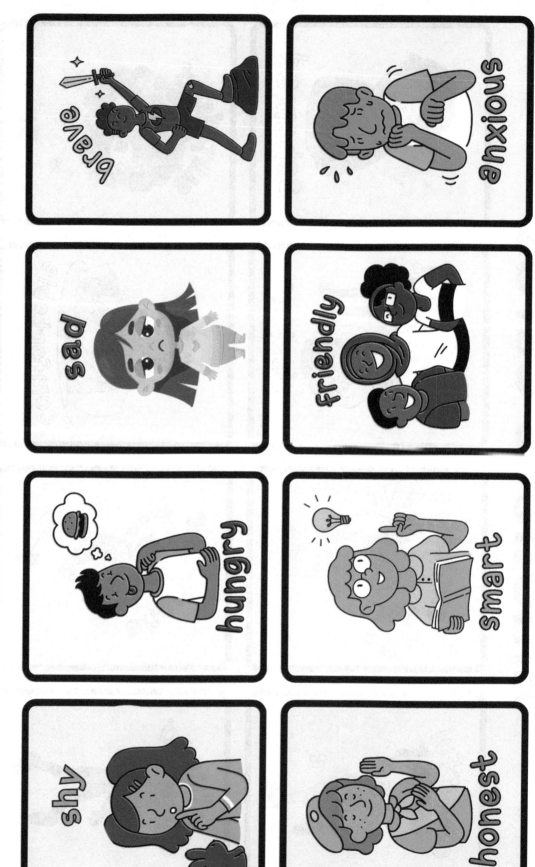

Emotions Cards

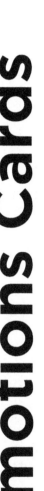

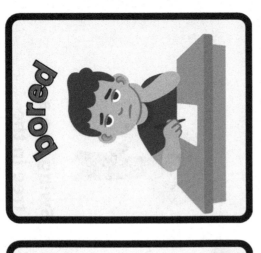

bored

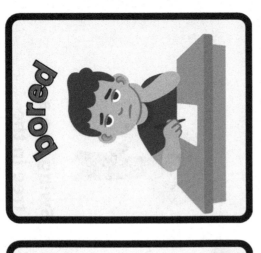

worried

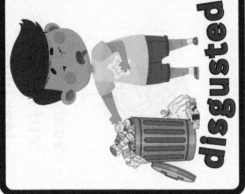

disgusted

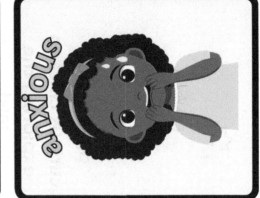

anxious

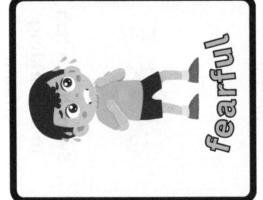

fearful

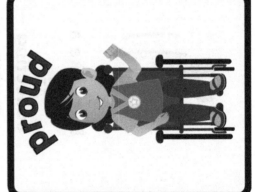

proud

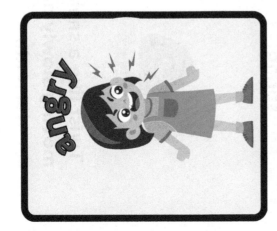

angry

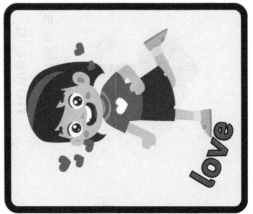

love

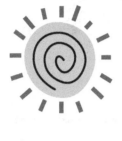

Radiate like the sun and shine a bright smile.

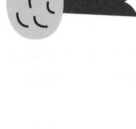

Swing like a tree in the wind.

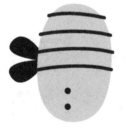

Peck like a curious chicken exploring the yard.

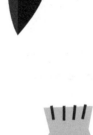

Soar like a bird in the clear blue sky.

Buzz like a bee collecting nectar.

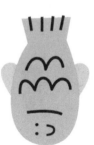

Swim like a fish in a sparkling stream.

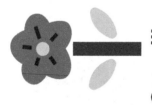

Grow like a flower in spring.

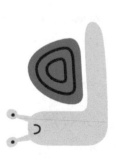

Twist like a snail moving slowly on its path.

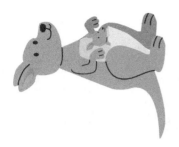

Stand tall and stretch like a mountain

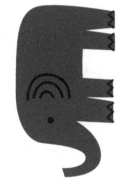

Crawl and roar like a lion.

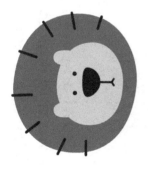

Stomp your feet and move your arm like a trunk.

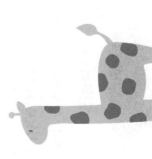

Hop like a kangaroo.

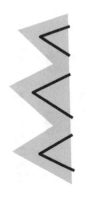

Walk tall like a giraffe on your tip-toes.

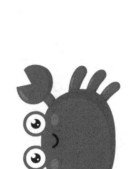

Flap your arms gently like a butterfly.

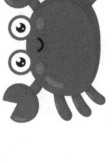

Walk on hands & feet like a crab.

Hop like a frog. Catch a bug with your tongue.

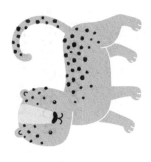

Sprint with short bursts like a cheetah.

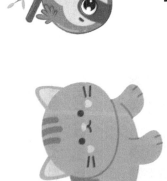

Move very slow like a sloth.

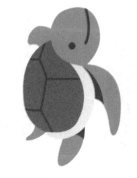

Swim through the ocean like a sea turtle.

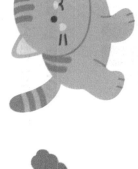

Walk gently like a kitten.

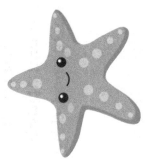

Stretch your arms and legs slowly like a starfish.

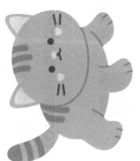

Crawl on your arms and legs to play like a pup.

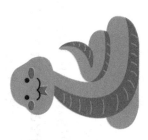

Slither on your belly like a snake.

Gallop or trot like a horse in the field.

FEELINGS THERMOMETER

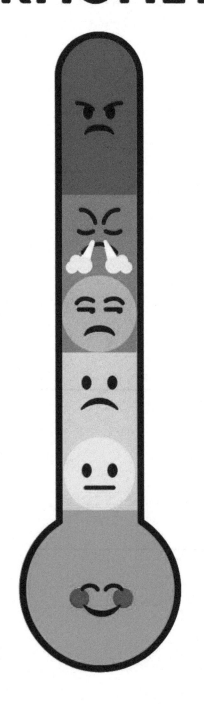

FEELINGS THERMOMETER

Color the thermometer to represent your emotion.

Write a word to describe how you are feeling.

Draw a face to show your emotion.

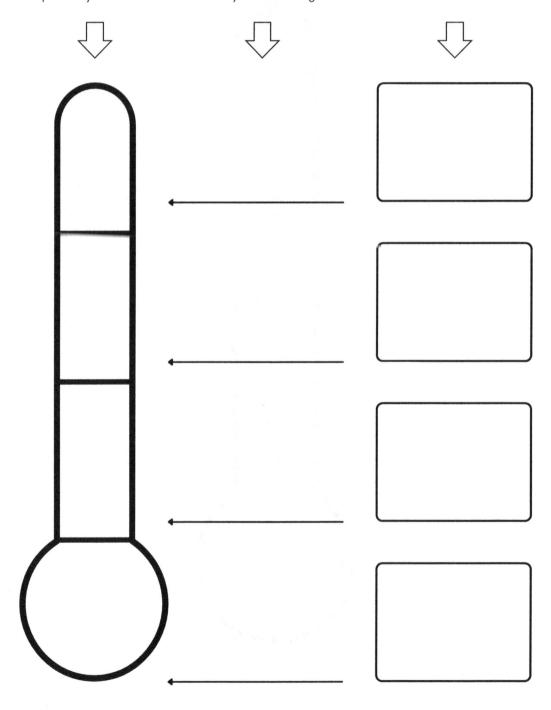

EMOTIONS VOLCANO

Emotions are like a volcano. They can sometimes puff smoke often like a steamy volcano. In this way, we let out our feelings little by little. Other times, we keep our emotions inside and then erupt when we do not expect it.

Anger lets us know something is going on in our body

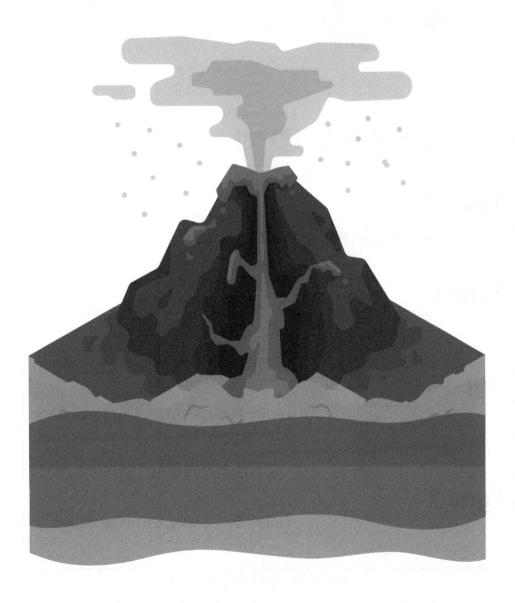

Stool Chart

Type 1

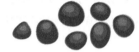

Separate hard lumps, like nuts or rabbit droppings. Hard to pass.

Type 2

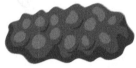

Sausage-shaped but lumpy. Like a tight bunch of grapes.

Type 3

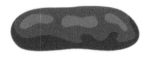

Like a sausage but with cracks on its surface. Like corn on the cob.

Type 4

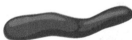

Like a sausage or snake. Soft and smooth.

Type 5

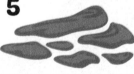

Looks like chicken nuggets. Soft blobs with clear-cut edges.

Type 6

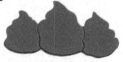

Looks like porridge. Fluffy pieces with ragged edges. A mushy stool

Type 7

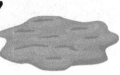

Looks like gravy. Entirely liquid.

Based on the Bristol Stool Chart

Made in the USA
Coppell, TX
10 October 2024